DisElderly Conduct

*Dis*Elderly Conduct

The Flawed Business of Assisted Living and Hospice

Judy Karofsky

A policy-driven memoir intended to promote public discussion of issues vital to the development of healthy, socially just communities for the elderly

New Village Press • New York

Published in the United States by New Village Press
bookorders@newvillagepress.net
www.newvillagepress.org
New Village Press is a public-benefit, nonprofit publisher
Distributed by NYU Press

Paperback ISBN: 978-1-61332-267-3
Hardcover ISBN 978-1-61332-268-0
eBook Trade ISBN 978-1-61332-269-7
eBook Institutional ISBN 978-1-61332-270-3

Library of Congress Control Number: 2024951630

Dialogue and events are from memory, personal notes, and electronic records. Certain identifying characteristics were altered to protect privacy and locations.
There are no federal rules or guidelines covering assisted living, but individual states have adopted laws for licensing and management. Excerpts from Wisconsin's Administrative Code are included as references.
The federal Medicare program establishes a baseline for hospice services, and states may adopt more stringent requirements.

Contents

Background

We are currently experiencing the future of eldercare that was predicted in the early years of the twenty-first century: Baby boomers are entering their eighties, and Generation Xers—in their forties and fifties—are making long-term care decisions for boomer parents.[1]

While becoming today's adult children, Gen Xers experienced historic economic events—from the dot.com bubble and September 11 to the housing boom and Great Recession of 2007–2009. Then came climate change, the COVID-19 pandemic, supply-chain dislocations, staffing issues, and rapid inflation. Over the course of two decades, the Gen X cohort matured into today's knowledgeable—sometimes wary—consumers and are now selecting living and care solutions not only for their parents but also for themselves.

In addition, family separations, divorces, and decisions to remain childless have led to a predicted cohort of "solo agers," who remain without family assistance and are making their own

---

1. The U.S. population age sixty-five and over grew from 2010 to 2020 at the fastest rate since 1880 to 1890 and reached 55.8 million, a 38.6 percent increase, in just ten years. United States Census Bureau, www.census.gov.

decisions. Many of these decisions are changing the landscape of the elderly housing environment.

For two decades that were characterized by demographics tilting toward an older population, sweeping changes occurred in the long-term care industry. At the beginning of the century, seniors housing was predominantly a local family and small business operation. Now ownership has evolved from on-site and local to regional and national. Today's mix offers over-fifty-five "enhanced active adult" housing, plus a smorgasbord of congregate spaces—independent living, assisted living (with or without memory care), and skilled nursing.

This book does not discuss *skilled nursing homes,* where the federal government makes and enforces the rules, and patients receive 24/7 nursing care or short-term postoperative rehabilitation. Nor does the discussion focus on *independent living,* where residents come and go at will, manage their own health care and medications, shop for and cook their own meals (usually, one meal per day is provided), and even continue to drive.

This book illuminates *assisted living facilities*—attractively landscaped complexes advertised as "homelike alternatives"—providing rooms, activities, meals, and limited health attention for those who are still mobile and not in need of skilled nursing. *Memory care* is the subset of assisted living that provides additional security to prevent wandering and offers specialized programming for those suffering from Alzheimer's disease or dementia. Assisted living and assisted living/memory care facilities are not regulated by the federal government but receive varying levels of oversight from state agencies.[2] They presently outnumber skilled nursing home sites.[3]

---

2. Assisted living or memory care facilities and any group home for adults that houses five or more unrelated residents, who receive care or treatment beyond room and board, are licensed in Wisconsin as community-based residential facilities (CBRFs).

3. "According to the Centers for Disease Control and Prevention (CDC) 2024 data, the U.S. contains 15,600 nursing homes with over 1.7

• • •

Depending on location, amenities, and assistance needs, assisted living bills can range from five thousand to twenty thousand dollars per month. Although qualifying for certain individual income tax deductions, assisted living and memory care rents and fees are *not* covered by Medicare. When hospice personnel certify that someone is within six months of death, hospice services can be initiated. The U.S. Medicare program will reimburse the cost of end-of-life care and supplies to participating hospice agencies— not to dying patients, next of kin, or other responsible parties.

Upon admittance, assisted living staff nurses examine residents to assess required care levels and fee ranges. Whether articulated by points or categories, the calculations are functions of time: A facility will be compensated for the number of staff hours allotted for care (bathing, dressing, nursing attention, feeding). Except in facilities where costs are guaranteed to remain constant, fees will keep pace with decisions about advancing health needs that are unrelated to inflation.

In recent years, as both the nationwide proliferation of new and expanded facilities and the impact of the pandemic placed extra burdens on assisted living staff, facilities turned to itinerant caregivers— employees of intermediary staffing agencies—and care costs increased. These costs are normally not absorbed by the community or management but are passed on to residents and their families.

Aside from federal financial assistance allocated during the pandemic period, assisted living payments continue to come from personal or family resources—pensions, Social Security, individual retirement accounts, and private savings or investments. Residents

million total licensed beds." AARP, www.theseniorlist.com. Meanwhile, "There are approximately 30,600 assisted living communities with nearly 1.2 million licensed beds in the U.S." American Health Care Association, www.ahcancal.org.

tend to represent the middle market—financially capable of paying for rent and care but neither superrich nor qualified for Medicaid support. As residents' ages advance and their prognoses decline, Medicare reimbursements to hospice organizations alleviate some end-of-life cost burdens—but only for limited periods of time.

The relationship between assisted living facilities and hospice organizations can be deceiving. "Half of all Americans now die in hospice care. Easy money and lack of regulation transformed a crusade to provide death with dignity into an industry rife with fraud and exploitation."[4] Patients certified as being within six months of death forgo curative care but receive medications to address pain and discomfort, nurses' attention (usually with twenty-four-hour phone coverage), diet monitoring, incontinence and mobility supplies (including wheelchairs), nonnursing attention for showers and skin care, and visits from community volunteers.

Medicare reimburses hospice agencies at a set rate per patient per day and requires periodic examinations to monitor the six-months-until-death limit. Patients and their families benefit by having medications and supplies delivered without charge. Assisted living or memory care facilities benefit by having certain activities removed from their purview; generally, they do not reduce the monthly charges or credit patients and responsible parties for cost savings.

Hospices, whether organized as for-profit or nonprofit, are businesses that employ marketing teams and practice image control. Although they reflect our human desire for death with dignity, their participation is conscribed by Medicare's rules for their compensation. They accept charitable donations that are frequently substantial and often publicized, but the federal government remains actively engaged in writing the rules and regulations.

---

4. Ava Kofman, "Endgame: How the Visionary Hospice Movement Became a For-Profit Hustler," *ProPublica* (copublished with *The New Yorker*), November 28, 2022.

*   *   *

Following the Recovery Act of 2009 and the restoration of the housing market, seniors became more willing to sell their homes and consider alternative living situations—either in their own communities or near relatives and children who could oversee their care. Demand increased for assisted living facilities that promised reliable, professional help with their daily lives. Without the buy-in common to independent living, month-to-month leases increased the possibility that residents could leave, but increasing frailty, need, and family inertia mitigated the risk.

As calculations of financial feasibility became more attractive, assisted living ownership expanded from individuals and partnerships to national franchises and corporations—both nonprofit and for-profit. Larger holdings have led to economies of scale that optimize marketing and operations and incentivize investment by real estate investment trusts (REITs), pension funds, labor unions, and private equity firms.

A common perception is that older people and their families can make residential care choices from an array of locations and service categories. The reality is that alternatives and opportunities slip by with time and age, and each person—or decision-maker— faces options limited by the stage of physical ability and health acuity at the precise moment of need. There may be choices *within* categories of seniors housing but rarely *between* categories.

Planning to enter either age-restricted communities or independent living is an ongoing lifestyle discussion, but the decision to enroll in assisted living or memory care is unlikely to be either gradual or gentle. People who require help with daily activities and health care can remain at home with partial to full-time family or professional assistance, remain in independent living (if the facility allows and has space for health aides), or enter assisted living.

Moves to assisted living are event-driven—often with the knowledge and approval of medical personnel. Families and advocates are called upon to make decisions in their weakest, most emotional moments. Now, more than ever, they should be aware that they'll be challenged by organizational changes, new medication procedures, remote care, and rising fees.

Despite decades of new construction, we still do not have the capacity to meet projected demand. In light of perpetual budget debates and the changes that are occurring in our federal government, Medicare will remain a pawn that will affect hospice services. Only certain remarkable families are prepared to care for aging loved ones at home. Our profit-driven eldercare models are deficient, and we lack the motivation to support our demographic future.

• • •

When my mother progressed in age and her strength declined, she advanced through five distinct senior living environments: an over-fifty-five retirement community, independent living, assisted living (*six* different facilities), memory care, and skilled nursing. My attention here is on the period after she suffered a stroke and required help with common tasks—her difficult days in assisted living and, eventually, assisted living with hospice involvement.

An adult daughter accompanying her aging mother along the confusing, frequently defective path of assisted living and hospice, *I was already in my seventies.* At the time of her passing, our national long-term care system for our most frail citizens failed us both.

Prologue

For those asking questions about the American system of eldercare, my mother's story presents a cautionary tale.

Lillian Deutsch (born Cowan) was the oldest of three children. When she was eleven, her mother (my grandmother) died of a self-induced abortion. Because the Commonwealth of Massachusetts wouldn't allow my grandfather to rear his three children, my mom, her brother, and her sister became foster children—often living in separate homes.

To stabilize his family, my grandfather sold everything he owned and took his children back to England, from where he'd emigrated—and where his brother was a headmaster of schools, in Manchester. My mother was prepared and eager to live in a new country. She told me about the Cunard Line ship, and she talked about England her whole life—although she'd never been there.

When the four travelers arrived at the port of Liverpool, the authorities refused to admit them. My grandfather was, by then, a U.S. citizen; it was the beginning of the Great Depression, and he didn't have a job. We'll never know, but the fact that they were a Jewish family—the family name had recently been changed from

Cohen to Cowan—was likely the deciding factor. After days of arguing, they were sent back to the United States in the hold of the vessel—steerage. Even when the ship stopped at Halifax, Nova Scotia, they were not allowed to disembark.

After returning to Lowell, Massachusetts, and eventually moving to Boston, my young mom begged to keep house for her father and succeeded in convincing the Commonwealth that they could all live in one house, even while she was still in high school.

• • •

The year I graduated from college, my mother walked into the home office of New England Telephone and Telegraph (AT&T), located in downtown Boston. She told the receptionist she wanted a job interview and that they simply had to hire her. She spent her career in advertising, winning awards for national ads for the Yellow Pages. At her retirement dinner, I heard repeatedly how unusual it was for a woman—a Jewish woman—to reach her corporate rank.

Wherever she landed, my lively and pleasant mom became the center of attention, dressed in designer outfits from Filene's Basement, shiny jewelry, and hats. She and my father retired to Florida, where she lived for almost twenty-five years. After my father died, she developed a relationship with her dancing partner—a nationally known magician. They traveled to New York and Hawaii, and to magic conventions from Milwaukee to Las Vegas. My mother became president of her local women's social organization, and she began to perform stand-up comedy.

• • •

On New Year's Day, 2006, I was studying with my Sunday-morning Talmud group when I received a phone call from my mother's neighbors. My eighty-seven-year-old mom was in the hospital, where she'd been driven by friends after celebrating New Year's Eve at the clubhouse in their gated retirement community.

I lived almost fifteen hundred miles away. I called the hospital and confronted our first information barrier: I was a legal stranger. I said, "I'm her daughter—her only child!" I waited until I could talk to my mom directly. She said she had pneumonia. Interdependent, rather than independent, my mother relied on a support network of close relatives and neighbors to drive her home, but we knew we had to make a permanent change.

My mom selected a realtor, and within weeks, we sold her house, car, and most of her furniture to the first family who came to view the house. The one-story home was attractive and well maintained, but we had no idea that the amount she received would be the highest paid in her community in 2006, and—due to the real estate bubble—for several years to come.

In February, I flew to Florida, and my daughter flew south from New York to meet me. Fortunately, my mother was well organized—everything was neatly sorted and labeled. Unfortunately, she'd stocked up on paper goods and cleaning supplies as if Y2K was threatening to return.

My daughter and I started in one corner of my parents' dream retirement home and worked our way through the garage, two bedrooms, two bathrooms, porch, kitchen, living room, den, and dining room. We sorted, discarded, recycled, and packed.

Three weeks later, I returned to Florida, and the real work began. I taped a roll of white paper to the master bedroom door and created an artful list with a felt tip pen, starting with "Meet with packers and movers" and ending with "Say good-bye to relatives and neighbors."

● ● ●

Because I'd assisted in the development of, and researched issues in, seniors housing, I assumed I knew how to ask questions about food, activities, and care—the basic components for a stable long-term care living situation. But after visiting several locations, we chose proximity—the common fallback for family decision making. My mother moved to an independent living apartment in a continuing care retirement community (CCRC), mostly because it was close to my home.

For the following seven years, my mom was a participating member of my adopted city, and I had someone who shared my adventures. She joined me on business trips, we went to the theater and opera, and we visited my daughter on Long Island and my uncle in Delaware.

Sometimes, I was overwhelmed by the demands of one-on-one attention: We never missed a thrift store, but we also visited every type of medical specialist. After living away from each other for so long, I could barely plan a day without including my mother. One evening, when I told her I had no life, she responded, "You have no lights?"

● ● ●

When my mother was in her mid-nineties, the chaplain of her CCRC invited her to share in weekly meditation. She started to attend the peaceful hour-long sessions that were led by a retired nurse, and before long, I joined in. One Friday, my elder daughter—who worked three blocks away—agreed to meet us. We would have a three-generation meditation. My daughter was a few minutes late, but my mom didn't show up at all.

After the hour passed, I saw my mother walking toward the mediation space—a secluded chapel room, adorned with a stained-glass window. My mom was surprisingly difficult to understand—or believe. She said, "I fell asleep on the floor and had trouble standing up." I said, "We really missed you." The incident was strange but not alarming. I thought my mother might have become distracted somewhere else in the building and didn't want to confess what she'd *really* been up to, or, perhaps, she *had* taken a nap . . . but, why on the floor?

A few weeks later, I received a call reporting that my mom had attended another meditation session, at the end of which she remained still—not responding to voice or touch. Someone in the facility office had already dialed 911.

I hurried to my car and drove to the parking lot at the rear of her building. My mom was on a stretcher, being wheeled through the open doors of an emergency medical services van. She was smiling, looking alert, and chatting with the young technicians! At that point, she couldn't be released from the ambulance, so I followed the vehicle to a nearby emergency room. We spent the afternoon waiting while the medical staff ordered and ran tests, and we left without a specific diagnosis.

Thus began a series of monthly or bimonthly ER visits. After the third or fourth trip by emergency conveyance, I started to drive my mom in my own car. Someone would call me to say she was unresponsive, I'd rush to meet her, and we'd endure one more day in the hospital.

Physicians began to refer to the incidents as transient ischemic attacks (TIAs), or ministrokes. The events didn't seem to have lasting effects, other than exhaustion—for me as well as for my mom. After twenty-four to forty-eight hours, she was back to her usual self—dressing in colorful clothes, following national politics, joining in social activities, and sharing witty remarks.

I didn't consider what might come next. I didn't know that the incidents would become more debilitating and affect my mother's ability to live independently. Except for recording the timing in my own records and including them in her medical notes, we never mentioned the lost days, and she didn't seem to remember the details.

● ● ●

On a warm Wednesday evening at the end of July 2013, my mom and I sat on a metal park bench, listening to a community orchestra concert, while my two granddaughters sat on the curb. Someone passed out red balloons, and the two preteens held them and giggled. The scene was idyllic: a summer night, perfect for people watching, with light classical music playing nearby. As her friends from independent living passed by, my mother said to all, "This is my family." The picture remains in my mind, in vivid color—the last evening my mom would be healthy and stable.

The day after the concert, my mom called to say she'd lost her prescription sunglasses. I thought she said she'd been shopping at Walgreens, so I hurried to the store. No glasses. Then, she said she'd lost them at Target, and that someone had talked to her about dropping a lot of items. She was confused—and confusing me—but I didn't connect the dots. I called and visited Target, to where her facility often bused the residents—but no sunglasses.

In the late afternoon, my mom began complaining of back pain and decided to return to bed. From that moment—amid highly anticipated summer days—until the end of her life, my mother became increasingly dependent, and I devoted more time to her care.

• • •

I began visiting every night and organizing pills for the next day; I helped with supper and eased her into bed. My mom slept a lot, but every morning when I arrived in her kitchen, I could see that she'd washed and dried the dishes and wiped the counter. Even in pain, my mother remained the willful child who'd cared for her father and siblings. She said, "I don't know" when I asked how the kitchen had become so clean. My delightful companion had another side: She was obsessively compulsive—insisting on being independent and helpful when she really wasn't.

After a long week, several calls to her private physician, and multiple doses of Tylenol, my mother agreed to visit her geriatric clinic. I borrowed a wheelchair from the adjacent health unit and wheeled my mom out to my car.

Once we arrived at the doctor's office, the same person who'd been in bed for several days started pacing in the small examination room, trying to relieve the pain in her back. She could not sit down. The doctor reviewed her medical records for possible (never diagnosed) sciatica. We talked about increasing her Tylenol intake, and I remember the exact moment when he looked at me and asked if I'd agree to trying oxycodone. I threw up my hands and said, "Sure." I was losing control and falling into medical confusion.

Within hours after my mother started taking the opioid painkiller, she began to totter and fall. "I feel drunk," she told me. Feeling increasingly responsible, I left several messages at the doctor's office over the next two days. I asked, "Are we giving her too much oxy? Should we cut back?" (Yes, of course, we should cut back.) By midweek, my mother was so constipated that I stopped the oxycodone and tried an array of over-the-counter cures for constipation—including her own standby, prune juice.

• • •

Wednesday, September 4, 2013, was the first evening of the Jewish New Year, Rosh Hashanah, a High Holiday. During the previous decade (even before she'd relocated from Florida), my mom joined me for High Holiday services. She was part of the small congregation—warmly received and accepted.

Now I attended evening services without her. The next day, I left her napping with my little dog while I met friends for lunch in a home about ten minutes from my mom's apartment. She said, "You should go. I'm comfortable in my own bed." I made certain she had access to her walker and left.

I enjoyed the respite and familiar faces, scattered through a neatly landscaped yard on a sunny afternoon—but I stayed fifteen minutes too long. When I arrived back at my mom's, she was face-down on the floor, perpendicular to her bed—lying in her own body waste.

I didn't know if my mother was embarrassed or incapacitated, but she was quiet. I shook off my shoes, stripped down to my underwear, and lifted my mom from the mess on the pale green carpet that we'd selected for her bedroom.

As I brought her walker closer, I could imagine how my mother might have reached for the walker when she was leaving her bed and probably hadn't locked it, so it propelled her toward the wall—pulling her to the floor. I directed my mom into her bathroom and we both undressed and stepped into her shower, where I cleaned her off.

• • •

When my mom left Florida, nearly seven years earlier, in the spring of 2006, we sold almost all her large belongings to snow-birds from New York State. We bought new furniture for her independent living apartment from an upscale furniture store: a brown-and-black tweed sofa, a coordinating dark red chair, an attractive iron bed, and half a dozen accent pillows.

I always thought I'd sleep in her living room—maybe many times—but I didn't know when it would be, or for how long. That night, after cleaning my mom and deciding we were done with oxycodone and all laxatives, my dog and I slept on the tweed sofa. I was exhausted, but I tried to stay alert.

At about 2:30 A.M., I heard a loud crash. The sound came not from my mom's bedroom, but from her bathroom. She'd left her bed and tried to negotiate the short hallway to the toilet.

Once again, I found my mother on the floor. The walker was pushed aside, and I guessed she'd tried to stand up from the toilet and thrust herself forward before she found her balance. Infuri-atingly, but not surprisingly, she said, "I didn't want to bother you."

In the morning, I decided to drive my mom to the emergency room—she was an elderly woman who'd sustained a potentially serious fall. I couldn't see any marks on her head, and she could stand and walk, but a wide area on her right buttock was starting to turn black-and-blue.

Something was wrong. My mother was not talking clearly. Because her smile was still symmetric, the examining physician said she didn't look like she'd had a stroke, but I knew she was failing the diagnostic tests. When the doctors asked her to touch her index fingers together, she struggled and missed, yet the neurology team said the motor weakness was because she was ninety-five years old.

Late in the afternoon, after I reminded the staff that my mother hadn't eaten breakfast, an attendant delivered a plastic container of applesauce. I watched my mom struggle, and I videoed her as she tried to spoon food into her mouth—with the spoon upside down.

The neurologist and hospitalist returned and said the slurred speech and manual clumsiness were the results of oxycodone. I said, "She hasn't taken the drug for the last two days." The neurologist started to calculate the half-life of oxycodone for a ninety-five-year-old woman. I felt like they were intentionally disregarding me—as if I were the child of a suspected heroin addict. I made several phone calls to stay in touch with the nurse and Personal Care Provider (PCP) at my mom's geriatrics clinic only a half mile away. When that clinic closed for the day, I was left alone without help or guidance.

Meanwhile, the doctors making decisions in the ER (the hospitalist and neurologist) insisted my mother couldn't be admitted to the hospital for observation. The hospitalist said, "A hospital is a terrible place for an old woman. She could fall or pick up an infection." A social worker joined the discussion. The hospitalist said they couldn't hold my mom because Medicare wouldn't pay if her hospital stay lasted fewer than three nights. The doctor looked at me and said, "It could cost you two thousand dollars." I said, "She's my mother!" He walked out.

. . .

I needed help. I needed someone on my side—a pair of professional ears. On Friday afternoon, Shabbat and the second day of Rosh Hashanah, I called the personal line of the social worker at Jewish Social Services (JSS). I'm not sure why she answered the phone, but she said she'd meet us at the hospital. By that time, there was nothing to do but proceed with the slow, detailed discharge process.

I wanted my mom to stay in the hospital, but I wanted to leave the emergency room as soon as possible. Neither my mom nor I had had any food. I wandered blindly into the cafeteria, which was already shutting down for the night.

I couldn't concentrate on meal choices. When I returned to the room where my mom was, with a plastic serving tray holding hot soup and bagels, she was sitting up—dressed to leave—and the discharge papers were ready for me to sign. I left the cafeteria choices uneaten and began to gather my mother's belongings. Our social worker promised to follow us.

I had no plan. I knew my mother was weak and disoriented, but I had no clue what was wrong with her or how I'd care for her over the weekend. As I was walking out of the room, pushing my mom in a wheelchair, one of the ER nurses looked at me and said, "You really wanted her to stay in the hospital, didn't you?" I said, "Well, yes, thank you. I did." (Weeks later, I bumped into a neighbor—a transplant surgeon—in a coffee shop. When I told him about the conversations in the ER, he suggested I contact the patient relations office and discuss the hospitalist, the neurologist, and the social worker's responsibility for a hospital readmission. I filed a complaint, as he suggested, and I tried to place a call to the director of the hospital but was derailed by the receptionist. By then, I was too distracted to pursue the matter.)

Finally, with my exhausted and disoriented mom in the passenger seat beside me, and the social worker from JSS following us, we drove to my mom's independent living apartment. On a Friday evening, I didn't know how to provide care or coverage for my mom. I also didn't know what was wrong with her or what could possibly happen next.

While driving, I called a friend who'd recently undergone surgery for a broken foot. Frustrated because the hospital had offered no help or suggestions, I asked her to brainstorm about what we needed and who could provide help.

My resourceful friend said she had a phone number for a woman entrepreneur who'd recently started a home-care agency. I called that number, once from my car and again when I was back in my mother's apartment and could think more clearly.

We'd barely survived one day since I returned from the warmth of a friend's home, after celebrating the blessings of the New Year, now dragging two tired bodies back to my mom's apartment. We hadn't eaten any food, and the ominous purple blotch on my mother's buttock was deepening and spreading.

The woman with the new care business said she could come meet us, even on a Friday night—or we could wait until Saturday morning. I needed to breathe and recalibrate; I chose the following morning. The social worker suggested that I sleep in my mom's bed overnight. I resisted, but she was right: I'd spent the previous night on the couch—asleep until I heard the loud crash in the bathroom.

I found soup in my mom's overstocked kitchen cabinet and fell asleep on her double bed—the beautiful iron bed we'd chosen and assembled for her life in independent living. My little dog slept between us. The second day of the Jewish New Year observance became the day we began a new intergenerational existence.

• • •

The social worker returned early on Saturday morning. While she stayed with my mom, I went to the independent living dining room to take advantage of a new weekend buffet service. I selected eggs and sweet rolls and was trying to balance cups of coffee on a tray when one of the first workers my mom had met and befriended, years before, came running after me to say I could no longer remove dishes from the dining room.

I said I had no intention of keeping any dishes. She said, "No." I had no warning about this policy, and I didn't have patience or energy for new rules. As she was still a resident of independent living, my mom was paying for a certain amount of monthly food service and gracious dining. I expected to be billed for our simple breakfasts.

I walked out with the institutional white plates, and the worker came trailing after me. I said I'd report her. (I hadn't the time or energy to follow through with a complaint to the very people who had instituted the change.) Other residents in my mother's building were gathering to stroll to the nearby Saturday farmers' market, and I longed to join them.

• • •

The first person in our eventual stream of helpers arrived after breakfast. I was inexperienced, but I believed she'd know how to take over as our caregiver and caretaker. She told us her fee was twenty-five dollars per hour. I had no idea how many hours were in a full day of caring or how long our needs would last, but I signed up. I needed someone to take charge—and she did.

Our new assistant said, "Everyone who cares for your mother will be a member of my family." She assured me that no one would begin to assume duties before they'd met us. My tired mom said she understood that members of a family would become her care team and said, "That's a relief." I slowly processed the scope of our roles: I would retain no responsibility beyond dispensing daily pills. My mother's job was to get well.

I received a list of items to purchase. Apparently, we needed latex gloves, boxes of sanitary wipes, and a baby monitor. Also—since my mother required nourishing food—we had to prepare a hearty chicken stew. Shopping list in hand, I drove to the nearest Target—glad to be alone and relieved to be out of my mom's apartment for a while.

I was living in two homes, and my mom's had become unfamiliar and overpopulated. I started to suspect that the entrepreneur's business came before my mom's needs. She gestured for quiet when she was on the phone with potential clients or members of her family—even as my mom asked for help to the bathroom. And, although the chef ate eagerly, the chicken stew contained unfamiliar spices that neither my adventuresome mom nor I was prepared to try.

As I watched my mother become more subdued, she seemed to disappear within her own surroundings. The caregiver decided to call her *Lilly*—not her name—and created visions about trips we'd all take to Boston. She told my mom she loved her, and she told me that my mom would improve. I wanted to believe her, so I did.

* * *

Four years later, as I was writing these paragraphs, I finally decided to perform essential due diligence on the start-up caregiving business. I read that the enterprise was formed to help and charge people for housework and errands. From an article in a local business journal dated three weeks before I'd signed a renewable one-week contract with the young company, I discovered that the owner had five clients and one part-time employee.

Thanks to the distant and dismissive hospital staff, we had no diagnosis, no prognosis, and no care plan. A bewildered and forlorn daughter, I'd left the ER with my impaired mother on a Friday evening and, not surprisingly, I hadn't asked the right questions. I was dealing with something more serious than a drug overdose, and we needed *health* care, not *house* care.

Now we had unprofessional, nonmedical people staying with my mom over the weekend, and I tried to make their lives more comfortable, because, after all, they were our houseguests. My mom and I were both suffering—and her condition could only become worse.

• • •

Early Tuesday morning, while walking my dog toward my mother's apartment, I received a call from the anxious care-business owner. She reported that another family member (whom my mom had not met before) had been in the apartment all morning.

Apparently, my mother woke up uncooperative and was now unresponsive. Despite assurances that we'd meet every caregiver, someone unfamiliar had attempted to wake and feed my mom. I said I was close by and hurried to her building.

The caregiver had already called the emergency number, 911. (I knew that the independent living facility forbade random ambulance calls, because they wanted to initiate and supervise all emergency calls from the office.) Instead of taking the elevator, I raced up the stairs and hurried through the door.

I found my mom perched on a designer metal stool at the bright new eating space that we'd hired a private contractor to create and paint. (The remodeling project had been completed only a few days before.) My mother was leaning precariously to her left side, and feeding her breakfast was out of the question. I couldn't see the future that morning, but my mother would never sit in her colorful kitchen again.

My mom was drooling. She was so limp, she required support to remain on her chair, and she didn't know I was there. Within minutes, paramedics lifted her onto a stretcher. I left my dog in the apartment and climbed into the caregiver's car. This time, I requested a trip to *another* hospital, because I was still angry about the treatment and abrupt discharge from the ER only four days before.

I was certain the caregiver was driving the wrong way, but she was merely taking an alternate route—her route. I remember looking at my iPhone and repeating the date: September 10, 2013. I was certain this was the day my mother would die. I sent text messages to my kids and, grateful for the ride, I sat back and stopped thinking.

We were waiting at the hospital when the attendants wheeled my mom off the ambulance. My first guardian angel, the emergency room physician, said he could diagnose a stroke because they'd recorded depressed vital signs when my mother was en route. My ninety-five-year-old mother had suffered a major stroke.

• • •

I'm an only child. Over seven years earlier, I'd brought my mom fifteen hundred miles north. We'd been on our own, because I had no choice. I'd made all the appointments, reservations, and decisions. Four days before, I'd contacted a caregiving business, seeking help I couldn't define, and three days before, I'd met the owner and signed a one-week contract.

On that confusing, emotion-laden poststroke morning, there wasn't room for all of us. While the private caregiver clung to the emergency that was playing out before us, she was lurking in a gray area of confidentiality and Health Insurance Portability and Accountability Act (HIPAA) violations. But part of me was relieved by her persistent, unexpected presence, and I asked her to stay so I could retrieve my dog from my mom's apartment, return to my own house, and take a shower. I set out on a long, brisk walk.

When I drove back to the hospital, I stopped to buy Italian sandwiches for the caregiver and myself—she was still our houseguest, and I thought my mom would still want me to offer her food.

This time, there was no question about a hospital admission: My mom had already been transferred to an inpatient floor. When I entered the room, I was surprised and troubled to find that the caregiver had continued to call my mom the wrong name. *Lilly* was written on the room's whiteboard, and I could guess that *Lilly* was written in the patient's chart. My mother had never been *Lilly,* and it was no time to change her name. She'd been *Lil* and she'd been *Lillian.* I found a way to say thank you and wished my assistant a good day—I needed to take over.

• • •

Sometime during my mom's second day in the hospital, my second guardian angel appeared: The staff neurologist came to offer us a *deal.* He said he could ask to have my mother accepted into the hospital's ten-day stroke rehab program. I heard him say there'd be family-style dining and daily therapy sessions, but, for some reason, what I remember most clearly was that he said she'd be dressed in street clothes. I guessed that wardrobe was either very important or included as a teaser. But I had no idea what to do next, and I needed no teasing.

I knew I couldn't care for my mother by myself. Without the offer of the inpatient rehab program, I'd have been lost—I was lost anyway.

My mom moved to the hospital stroke floor the next day. For one long week, I helped her with every meal. I watched and listened as someone encouraged her to stand up and take steps with a walker. We'd never thought about a wheelchair, and didn't plan to own one, but someone signed us up for a wheelchair, which—under Medicare rules—we'd rent to own, and which would be sent home with her, although *home* was still an unspecified location.

I watched the staff show my mom how to write and use silverware. I attended a family meeting where someone handed out computer-printed descriptions of strokes, stroke causes, and stroke warnings. I tried to stay focused, but I was in frightening, uncharted territory.

As I left for home the first night, I noticed a form at the unit desk that appeared to be an application for visiting dogs, and I checked with the person at the main information kiosk near the hospital's exit doors. Yes! If I had proof of up-to-date vaccinations and a uniformed security officer could meet my eighteen-pound dog, Bacon would be allowed into the hospital.

Nothing could have helped my mom connect with her recovery plan as easily as my dog. He knew exactly what to do when I took him to her room early the next morning: He jumped on her bed—and he stayed.

One after the other, the days passed. When I left the stroke unit to buy food in the hospital cafeteria, I was keenly aware of events playing out one floor below—the busy maternity floor. Women came in; women and babies left. Couples came in; couples and babies left. Families came in . . . at all hours, every day, all week. Lives were changing one floor beneath us, and family life was beginning.

Because it was still September, we could sit outside on a sunny deck off the stroke unit, and I could help my mother eat al fresco. On Friday, we looked up and saw the private caregiver who'd promised, a few days earlier, that she'd return to visit my mom.

We chatted until the caregiver realized there were other stroke-affected families scattered at other patio tables. Without hesitation, she circulated and introduced herself to the remaining families—whom I barely knew. She left her business cards and said they could contact her if they needed help.

My mom, who'd suffered a major stroke, could still process what was happening and told me, "She just wants to be paid." Although the assistance lasted from Saturday morning until Tuesday's ride to the emergency room (three days), I received an invoice for the entire week.

My mom wanted the transaction to be over as quickly as possible. She looked at me and said, "Pay her whatever she wants." I'd signed a contract for one week's service, and there were no refunds. I wrote a check for two thousand dollars, the same amount the hospitalist had warned I might pay for medical care if they admitted my mother—as they should have—one week before.

One nearby family member complained, and the floor nurse approached the intruding caregiver and asked her to leave. She told her never to appear again—she'd been soliciting business at the hospital and was lucky to leave with just harsh words. In time, I brought the incident to the attention of my friend who'd made the referral on the confusing Friday evening, one week earlier. My friend said the caregiver had recently started her business and would have to learn about boundaries. I told myself I'd have to learn to establish boundaries of my own and start to ask questions—lots of questions.

● ● ●

Amid daily therapy, meetings, setbacks, decisions, and caring for both my mom's independent living apartment and my own house, I received visits from persistent hospital social workers. I'd met with their colleagues more than six years before, when my mom had a brief hospital stay after a ministroke. At that time, we arranged a temporary transfer to the health center connected to her long-term care complex.

No one was talking about a temporary placement this time: We had to locate a home for the rest of my mom's life—and decide how she'd receive care. The social workers' role wasn't to sift through assisted living facility options or help us anticipate future needs. Their assignment, from their employer—the hospital—was to facilitate my mother's exit from the stroke unit. Medical economics drove the discussion.

My mom was mobile but required constant watching. The stroke left her with core weakness that forced her body off balance and caused her to plop into a chair—rather than gracefully take her seat—and she seemed to have lost her basic sense of safety.

Our options included care in my own home (I could move to a more accessible home or apartment); I could have placed my mom in any area assisted living facility; or she could have returned to Florida—and I'd have accompanied her. I was the only person responsible, and I watched my patient every moment. I was making both major and minor choices, and I couldn't organize visits to alternate assisted living locations. What would I look for?

When the hospital social workers started talking about the assisted living section of my mother's existing CCRC I agreed— actually, I succumbed. I had no understanding of how the move would happen or what a complete change would occur in our lives.

● ● ●

One afternoon, when I visited the independent living apartment to retrieve fresh clothes for my mom, I met with the newly hired director of the assisted living program. He showed me two potentially available rooms: One was on the main floor, near the entrance and dining room, and didn't require elevator access. The other, on the lower floor, necessitated elevator trips, and was currently occupied. The director said the resident wanted to move to the room on the first floor, but if she decided not to move, my mother could have the more accessible room.

As I looked around, the assisted living section appeared worn, darkly furnished, and abandoned—reflecting what I guessed was a period of almost twenty years of reassigning spaces without an overall renovation. I wasn't inspired by what I saw—I knew my mom would be saddened by the atmosphere, and I anticipated being dejected along with her.

My mother still cared about her hair, clothes, and space, and she observed and commented on her surroundings. I asked if we could paint a few walls in the bedroom and bathroom before my mother moved in, and the director agreed—I could pick bright, cheery colors if I purchased the paint.

When he called to say the first-floor room was available, I knew we were locked in. I never investigated another assisted living facility in the area—never compared activities, meals, or care. My mom was recovering from a stroke in a nearby hospital, and I chose the most direct route: She moved down the hill and remained in her familiar housing community. On Friday, September 20, 2013, my mom announced her arrival "I'm here," she said. The assistant director of the assisted living wing responded, "Everyone ends up here."

Nowhere to Die

When my mother was one month shy of eighty-eight years old, I'd helped her move from her own home and gardens in Florida to an independent living apartment in a long-term care complex in my midwestern city. She'd clung to her independence for seven and a half years.

Now, when she required additional care, she became an occupant of community-based residential facilities (CBRFs) licensed by the state of Wisconsin to serve residents of advanced age and those with irreversible dementia or Alzheimer's disease. During the next four and a half years, as she became weaker from advancing age, vascular dementia, and a hip fracture, she moved back and forth between six different assisted living residences, in four municipalities, all within one county.

According to Keren Brown Wilson, the first written use of the term *assisted living* was in a 1985 proposal to the state of Oregon to fund a pilot study.

By 1988, assisted living was being used in presentations at professional meetings and in early trade publication articles. By 1991 . . .

27

many residential care facilities that offered or arranged care were calling themselves assisted living, and the study included assisted living as an explicit subset of residential care.

. . . [T]he early models of assisted living emerged in reaction to nursing facilities and a vision of a different way of bringing physical environments, care and service capacity, and philosophy together to offer a more desirable product to older people, many of whom were in or destined for nursing facilities.[5]

During biennial budget deliberations for 1994–1995, the Wisconsin legislature joined lawmakers in a handful of other states in adopting a requirement of homelike apartment settings for "assisted living" residences for people who could—or chose to—no longer live independently but did not require skilled nursing.

In Wisconsin, CBRFs are regulated under Chapter DHS 83, Wisconsin Administrative Code:

"Assisted Living Facility" is a term that encompasses . . . facilities licensed, certified, or registered by the Department of Health Services. All assisted living facilities combine housing with services to help people remain as independent as possible. . . .

A CBRF is a place where:

- five or more adults, not related to the operator or administrator,
- do not require care above intermediate level nursing care,
- reside and receive care, treatment, or services above the level of room and board, but that

---

5. Keren Brown Wilson, Ph.D. "Historical Evolution of Assisted Living in the United States, 1979 to the Present," *The Gerontologist* 47 (December 2007): 8–22.

- provides not more than three hours of care per week per resident.[6]

Once my mom's health forced her to relinquish her independent lifestyle, she lived in the following facilities:

1. The assisted living section of a nonprofit CCRC that included independent living, assisted living, and a skilled nursing/rehabilitation center

2. The assisted living floor of a private (franchised) assisted living/secure memory care CBRF

3. A secure memory care section within a private (corporate) CBRF/residential care apartment complex (RCAC)

4. A ubiquitous, freestanding private assisted living CBRF

5. A secure assisted living/memory care, private (franchised) CBRF

6. The assisted living section of a nonprofit CCRC, a community that included retirement housing, independent living, and memory care and had recently phased out its skilled nursing wing

Each facility was established and marketed as a healthy, safe home for elderly residents. Depending on amenities and care level, we paid between $5,100 and $12,000 a month. Many of our experiences were disappointing, and I can describe only the conditions we observed during the period when my mom was a resident of each home. Over time, the three essential components—food, activities, and care—may have been updated in some or all.

---

6. "Choosing an Assisted Living Facility," State of Wisconsin, Department of Health Services, Division of Quality Assurance, Bureau of Assisted Living, P-60579 (Rev. 09/2012), p. 2.

September 2013 to December 2014

First Facility

My mother began her assisted living saga nine days after she survived a major stroke. Bolstered by a hospital rehab program of physical, occupational, and speech therapy, she moved into a corner room in a new section of her long-term care complex.

While my mom lived in independent apartments we periodically visited the assisted living section for social calls with friends who'd relocated there, but the area—the entire program—remained unfamiliar. Although we'd transferred proceeds from the sale of a house in Florida to pay the entrance fee (redeemable upon exit) for the independent living section, and had paid monthly rent and food charges, my mother was not guaranteed a space in assisted living. Availability of a unit was one issue, but I learned that resident suitability was the ill-defined and illusive barrier to entry.

My mom became the first prospective resident for a new assisted living director. One afternoon, he appeared at the hospital, introduced himself, and sat in front of a computer, where he spent a couple of hours sifting through my mom's health records. He never discussed any issue with me, and I still have no idea what kept him staring at the screen, but he must have approved.

Alleging there'd be too much work for the staff nurse if there was a Friday move-in, the director insisted that my mom transfer on Thursday (a day before the stroke program at the hospital ended). Over my objection, he requested and implemented her early hospital discharge. I remembered his words many times after that week, when I watched families bring loved ones to the facility on Fridays, Saturdays, and even Sunday nights.

For what would not be the last time, I yielded to the illogical whim of authority. On an autumn Thursday morning, I participated in my weakened mom's discharge from inpatient care. She was transported via van and wheeled into her new home on the seat of the hospital wheelchair that we'd contracted to purchase. Because my mother still considered herself *able,* the sight of a wheelchair frightened her. Eventually, she'd own or rent several, but for the next sixteen months, she relied on a series of walkers. We tucked the dreaded hospital item behind her bedroom door.

Sadly, for motion-compromised residents like my mom, the seventeen-year-old assisted living section had become functionally obsolete. Residents lived longer, survived with more disabilities, and used more mobility aids than was predicted when the building was designed.

Planners at the long-term care complex's corporate headquarters—two thousand miles away—had focused on creating attractive public areas and apartments for *independent* living. They'd introduced upscale features to encourage older retirees to relocate to the congregate residence but had spent little effort on the *assisted living* and *memory care* wings, where most residents would eventually live. The independent living common area featured a full-sized movie screen and a modern sound system, but the small sitting area near my mom's new room offered only a small TV compromised by blurry images and unreliable reception. Complicated wayfinding, faded decor, and recycled couches lent a dated atmosphere to the space. The resulting ambience was uninviting and sad.

I began to receive weekly calls that my mom had fallen in her long, narrow bathroom. She was correct when she looked at me and said, "There's not enough room in the bathroom for both the walker and me."

A well-meaning physical therapist visited and tried to teach my mother to turn around and *back into* her bathroom—pulling her walker with her—but the recommended reverse action led to even more falls. I came to understand what a health columnist meant when she described an ageist attitude surrounding physical and cognitive decline—when observers and assistants respond as though "old people fall all the time and maybe they shouldn't be walking around."[7]

Precisely when my mom craved comfort and attention, the quality of amenities, activities, and food service declined. As she became dependent on her walker and her strength waned, we shortened our daily walks.

When autumn passed into winter, she became more and more confined—she missed the social activity and gathering spots in independent living. My mother really didn't know where to go—except to her own bedroom.

· · ·

In my initial research, I read that although a limited number of regulations govern assisted living facilities in Wisconsin, every facility is required to provide:

> . . . a living environment for residents that is as homelike as possible and is the least restrictive of each resident's freedom; and that care and services a resident needs are provided in a manner that protects the rights and dignity of the resident and that encourages the resident to move toward functional independence in daily living or to maintain independent functioning to the highest possible extent.[8]

I wrote email messages and sent letters to the management. We attended an individual care meeting with the assisted living director, where I asked what my mother and the other residents

---

7. Paula Span, "How Ageism Can Take Years Off Seniors' Lives," *New York Times*, April 26, 2022.

8. Wisconsin Administrative Code, Chapter DHS 83, "Community-Based Residential Facilities," Subchapter I—"General Provisions," DHS 83.01—"Authority and purpose."

were expected to do during their quiet hours, and I received a follow-up response that acknowledged my mom's frequent falls.

The director reported that they tried to generate ideas on how to engage her after breakfast—perhaps by detouring her from going back to her room. He suggested taking my mother to the sunroom or out on the patio. (In either location she'd most likely be left alone.) He said that he hoped to try this tactic, because "once Lillian goes back to her room, she is very unlikely to participate in a morning activity."

I did not respond, but if I had, I'd have suggested that the solution to my mother's boredom and inactivity was *not* parking her somewhere and leaving her unsupervised after breakfast. I could tell that my role as her activity coordinator was about to expand.

Another suggestion from the same meeting referred to my request that more than one staff member be assigned to resident lunch outings—for the safety of all. On an earlier field trip, my mom fell from the van to the sidewalk, while the activities director was helping another resident, who'd also slipped. Apparently, I'd said I'd be willing to join the outings, on occasion, because the staff was directed to send me an invitation!

And because this had become *my* issue and no one else's concern, I was told, "Staff are to encourage Lillian to try a larger variety of food in the dining room." I knew that encouraging her to *try* a larger variety was not a solution. Looking back, I realize the comment was both demeaning and ageist. Creating a more varied and appetizing menu would have been the answer.

The prevailing dismissive attitude mattered because my mom knew she was physically removed from—and forgotten by—her formerly supportive independent living community. She felt isolated and neglected, and she told me, "Nothing will ever change."

We were paying for care services and "a living environment for residents . . . as homelike as possible," which I knew my mom was not receiving. "We will never be able to satisfy you," the executive director of the retirement complex said at the end of one meeting. Clearly, the relationship was becoming adversarial.

On an official-looking sign, posted in the hallway, I read that there was an office of a state ombudsman for nursing homes—including assisted living facilities—and I started calling the listed number to ask questions about unmet expectations for my mother's daily life.

· · ·

My mom asked me why no one cared that wet mops were left standing in the hallway. They were not only unclean but unsafe, and they were an affront to a resident with burgeoning obsessive-compulsive disorder (OCD). Becca Levy, a psychologist and epidemiologist at the Yale School of Public Health, says that "ageism results in more than hurt feelings or even discriminatory behavior. It affects physical and cognitive health in measurable ways and can take years off one's life."[9]

In trying to extend and enhance her days, I'd unintentionally selected a space where my mom's comfort and sensibilities were being challenged, and I feared a serious fall. For undisclosed reasons, the director fired the nurse who'd been my mother's primary support and one of her guiding lights. He told me he had no plans to search for a replacement because he'd previously been in charge of a facility north of the city, and he said, "I ran it without a nurse."

My mom started reporting about residents who transferred to other places, and I realized we were not locked into a facility because of either its convenient location or its attachment to a former, familiar home in the independent living section. Because I longed to improve her outlook, I became willing to help my mother move, but I had no notion how a relocation could disrupt our lives.

---

9. Paula Span, "How Ageism Can Take Years Off Seniors' Lives." *New York Times,* April 26, 2022.

December 2014 to April 2016

Second Facility

After a year and three months in a space I thought would be her only such home, I helped my mother transfer to the assisted living floor of a year-old combination memory care/assisted living facility. Christmas trees were twinkling, and vases were filled with fresh flowers. When we entered the front door for her initial visit, the first thing she said was, "It's so clean here." Just like her three adult homes, including the one in which I grew up.

The facility's director, who had worked as a certified nurse assistant (CNA) in my mom's previous CCRC was eager to welcome new residents. Someone might have reviewed my mom's medical records, but the admissions process I recall was a reasonable, detailed discussion about fees and potential cost increases with future care needs.

Located on a corner lot, the new building featured short hallways with small bedrooms. Predictably, the director said, "But she won't be spending much time in her room." After two visits, I selected a recently vacated, slightly more expensive two-bedroom suite, originally intended for couples: Apartment 113. "Not a good number," my mother said.

Officially, she was renting only the bedroom, bathroom, and adjoining living room, and we were not charged for the second bedroom. My mom was confused by the extra door, and when we began storing equipment like a wheelchair and nebulizers there, she started referring to the disorganized space as her "garage."

In a welcome advantage over her initial assisted living space, the bathrooms and showers were more accessible. However, the awkward common areas were frequently rendered impassable by scattered wheelchairs, walkers, dining tables, and guest seating—especially for aging residents with physical limitations.

. . .

On the day we celebrated Martin Luther King, Jr., five weeks after entering the home where we'd transferred my mom because of my fear of her falling, my mother was discovered on the floor behind her bedroom door. (Her door opened in—toward the room—making the entrance dangerous if she was trying to leave while another person was trying to enter.)

Since her stroke, my mom had exhibited diminished balance and core strength, as well as a certain inability to assess her own weakness. When she fell, she may have been separated from her walker. In an instant—precisely as I was driving to visit her—an unwitnessed fall left my ninety-six-year-old mom with a broken hip, an accident that changed the course of our lives.

Reluctant to call an ambulance to the facility, the resident nurse contacted a mobile X-ray provider. I watched the facility's director help my mother limp to the bathroom two times, even as my mother clearly cried, "You're making matters worse."

Five hours after the fall, following a diagnosis by the mobile x-ray technician, my impaired mom was finally transported to an emergency room by ambulance. I will never understand the delay in action. As soon as the hospital's doctor administered morphine for her pain, I allowed myself to admit what had been happening all afternoon and evening. I remember a wave of nausea rising from my belly. I blamed myself and vowed never again to let my guard down. Moving ahead, I would have to remain alert and assertive.

. . .

Once stabilized, my mother underwent major surgery—with a few complications. In retrospect, she should have recuperated at a skilled nursing facility—one that offered a dedicated program of physical therapy (PT). We faced a classic assisted living dilemma: remain where she was living and arrange for visiting care or move to a location that offered on-site rehab services.

Because my mom had recently relocated and was both emotionally and physically fragile, acclimating her to a temporary home seemed unnecessarily disruptive. Also, we were motivated to return to her second assisted living accommodations because we were already paying rent to the facility. (The logic of the rent calculation was ill-conceived, because Medicare likely would have covered a stay in rehab.)

Hospital social workers started to ask about our plans. They couldn't make decisions for us, and I didn't have the time or energy to travel to the nursing/rehab facilities they mentioned. I wanted to stay with my mom. The nurse and director of my mother's current assisted living home both visited the hospital. My mom seemed happy to see them, and we all decided her preferred *home* was with them.

When they visited, the assisted living staff assured me that my mother could receive therapy in her accustomed setting, but I wasn't listening carefully enough to hear that the assistance would be provided by private therapists. I didn't understand that the building had no gym, exercise room, or rehab equipment. (Even now, as I prepare this book, I have a recurrent dream that there's a side door to the structure, and that it leads to a lap pool.)

Although I was frequently frustrated by my mother's wavering coordination and my inability to urge her along, I tried to assist the visiting therapists. I accompanied them as they led her to exercise in her room and attempt taking steps along the common hallway.

Now, I recall how my fear increased when the therapist scheduled a walk outdoors—on the hard sidewalk surface. I know the exact location where we all admitted we were not helping. I've accepted the reality that my mom's stroke robbed her of core strength and balance—if she'd regained mobility and independence, she might have continued to fall.

• • •

My mother never walked again. For her final three years, everything about our lives focused on mobility. I learned to transfer her into and out of dining room chairs, cars, and bathrooms, and I repeatedly sought the most comfortable and practical wheelchairs. Even with warm-weather walks around the suburban neighborhood, a nearby tennis center, and a nature trail, my mother's world shrank. The economical and efficient—but limited—interior floor space at the new, clean assisted living facility proved to be confining. My mom hovered in the common area, surrounded by activity and ambient noise that wasn't relaxing, and she impatiently sought relief. Other visitors told me that she began calling my name. My brave mother was waiting for me to show up with my dog.

• • •

Once her hands-on requirements increased, I had no choice but to devote additional hours to my mom's needs. When I wasn't on-site, I worried about random details of care. Not for the first time, I became aware of the essential role of assisted living CNAs. As at her previous residence, I was prepared to fill in and back up the staff, but almost every morning, when I arrived and asked how things were going, I received a dismissive one-word response from the people who'd presumably awakened, dressed, and fed her: "Good."

Gradually taking the day's inventory, I'd discover that my mother's linens were soaked; or her hearing aid batteries were lost in the sheets, because the aids had been left in all night; or her TV had never been turned off. And there was the constant state of alertness for ministrokes that occurred almost like clockwork, at six-week intervals, leaving my weakened mom noncommunicative and noncompliant for most of the day.

● ● ●

In April 2015, the assisted facility staff suggested my mother might be close enough to death to be eligible for medical services and regular visits from a local nonprofit hospice organization. One month later, we signed her up, but I still retained the role of *assistant* in her assisted living.

Even with 24/7 assisted living care, for which we continued to pay, and without thinking or worrying about long-term implications, I functioned as the bedtime caregiver. I washed my mom's face, removed her hearing aids, and changed her into a nightgown. Every night, I turned on a light TV program (although she really wanted to watch CNN news) and transferred her increasingly unstable body to bed. My dog and I both kissed her good night, and I drove home, exhausted and haunted by care lapses that could occur in my absence.

● ● ●

Despite other limitations, the laundry room at my mother's first assisted living place was clean and well-organized—ample for the floor on which she lived. But, sometime during the early weeks at her second home, I noticed that her clean laundry pile contained items belonging to other people: men's underwear, a nightgown that was too big for her, and single socks. Moreover, some of her shirts and pants were missing. Obviously, her laundry was being commingled with that of other residents.

The staff recommended that I label her clothes—like summer camp. I hesitated to write my mom's name on clothing, because I knew we'd eventually make donations to a charitable resale shop, and I didn't want her identity to be attached and legible.

Then I noticed that the staff were washing residents' belongings on a short cycle—recommended by the appliance manufacturer for newly purchased items. I calculated there might not be enough time in the day—or during one shift—to wash the belongings of everyone on my mom's floor in a single pair of household devices: one washer and one dryer. I knew that my mom's underwear and linens were frequently soiled, and I didn't want to think about the other residents' belongings.

Without hesitating, I reverted to the days when I'd been a stay-at-home mother of three: I bought two large laundry bags and began lugging dirty laundry home to my own basement. I followed a nightly ritual: prewash the soiled items and continue with the entire load of laundry—load, wash, and dry. Many afternoons, I folded laundry while my mother dozed or watched TV.

* * *

As she aged and her wardrobe became less fashionable, my mom remained recognizable for her hair bows. She loved the colors and variety. (In time, we buried her remains with a collection of rainbow-colored bows and distributed many to the family mourners at her funeral.)

One night, in her second assisted living dining room, I noticed my mother was wearing *two* hair bows. I asked about them and she told me there'd been a scuffle in her bathroom. She showed me how the male assistant, who was helping her get dressed, had fondled her breasts. She showed me exactly what he did, and I had no reason to doubt her. She'd never told or created a story like that before. She said, "He put a second bow in my hair to make light of what he did."

When I left the facility, I lingered in my car in the dark parking lot. I was numb, wondering, What, now? As is common in moments following unwanted sexual incidents, I wanted to warn other women—everywhere. I called my daughter, who'd recently worked as the state's prosecutor for violence against women. She said, "Call the local rape crisis center."

There hadn't been a rape per se, but I contacted the twenty-four-hour help line. Still in the dark, I received the good advice that I meet with the social worker from my mom's facility. Of course, there was none, but I remembered that a friend, a social worker, worked at the area Jewish Social Services. (This was not the same social worker who'd assisted us during a hospital visit two years earlier.)

Over the next week, my mom and I met with the social worker and (when my mother was ready) with the facility's director. My mother's story didn't change.

I assumed the care organization had procedures in place, and, at the minimum, they'd transmit a confidential report to the licensing authority (the state). I was disappointed, although not surprised, that nothing was said about the episode again. The aide was kept out of my mother's room, and within six weeks, the resident nurse told me he'd been fired—presumably after another incident. She said, "Don't ask any questions," and I didn't. It was only the first time I suspected a facility might prefer to hide rather than disclose an unseemly event like an unwanted sexual advance—or any other assault—and that there were no clear procedures for reporting to the state or to any other regulating authority. To this day, I remain proud of my mother's forthright courage.[10]

* * *

Soon after the incident with the male helper, my mom let me know that she'd begun to feel unrecognized, awkward, and out of place. She seemed to withdraw, and I began to understand that she felt

---

10. "Reporting sexual assaults, which has always been difficult for survivors, continues to re-traumatize victims and often perpetuates a culture of victim-blaming." *Seattle Times*, October 26, 2023.

confined both emotionally and physically. Her assisted living residence (her second) was carefully designed to fill a vacant and available corner lot. The building benefited from curb appeal but lacked adequate internal space. Ultimately, the efficient structure couldn't meet the needs of an aging resident confined to a wheelchair.

Not recognizing her limitations, my mother repeatedly tried to leave her bed, but she only managed to fall to the floor. Even with additional floor padding to soften her landing, we couldn't trust her to nap unless someone observed her. If we settled her in her reclining wheelchair in the common activity/dining area for increasingly long snoozes, she was bombarded by TV, conversation, and confusion.

Over and over, I wheeled my mom, with my dog on her lap, along two short corridors. She memorized the paintings on the walls and said, "We've been here already." Indeed, we had. I was as lost as she was. Proceeding without operating instructions or a roadmap, I began looking for a new living situation.

When a professional in the eldercare industry told me that two friends had recently moved a parent into a newly opened facility, I began searching for the address. I had an indirect connection with one of the adult children, and although our needs differed, I trusted that she'd make a sound decision. Sadly, the route to assisted living and memory care solutions is strewn with poorly researched and reactionary choices like mine.

April 2016 to June 2017

Third Facility

As we packed for my mom's third assisted living residence, the director of her second one asked me, "Do you think she'll be able to die there?" I wasn't thinking of death; I was thinking of extended days of contentment. Repeated moving was medically unwise and emotionally draining, but now that my mom was confined to a wheelchair, starting over in a larger facility—with well-designed rooms and both indoor and outdoor spaces to investigate—seemed therapeutic. My mom was my constant companion, and I wanted to capture more of her smiles.

Before she could enter her third facility, my mother needed to complete a pre-admission evaluation. I brought her to the site on a Sunday morning. One of the nurses, still dressed in the black suit, frilly print blouse, and heels that she'd worn to church (for which she apologized), sat in a small side office and reviewed my mom's list of meds, then asked if my mom could move out of her wheelchair. I assisted with the transfer—and that was the extent of the assessment. It cost us two thousand dollars.

Unfortunately, the quick evaluation provided no indication that the rest of move-in would be simple. We faced a unique obstacle: The third facility had no defined assisted living section. Designed as an RCAC, the building configuration allowed too much freedom for someone in my mother's stage of physical decline and wheelchair dependence.[11] Also, because we'd activated power of attorney documents for my mom's care during a clinic visit the previous year, the intake nurse determined that my mom could be housed only in the secure *memory care* wing (assisted living—with locked doors into and out of the unit). Thus, even though she was still alert for her years and not diagnosed as an Alzheimer's patient, my mother moved to memory care.

The state of Wisconsin limits nursing services to three hours a week for residents in assisted living facilities, and the same for those in memory care. Hearing that she'd receive no additional

---

11. RCACs consist of independent apartments for five or more adults, each of which has an individual lockable entrance and exit. RCACs cannot admit individuals who have an active power of attorney for health care or have been found to be incapable of recognizing danger. www.dhs.wisconsin.gov/regulations/health-residential.htm.

nursing attention, I told myself a memory program might engage my mother's interests and remaining capabilities. She was not a flight risk—not in her wheelchair—but I believed that customized activities in a memory care setting could be stimulating. I had no guidebook, and I was tired of researching new situations and hiring movers. For the third time, we made a commitment to a new eldercare model.

• • •

On my mother's first evening in her new residence, the main dining room was filled with music, visitors, and a western-themed buffet celebrating the facility's third anniversary. I was certain we'd hit the motherload of abundant care. Besides being located near a city park, family restaurants, and a coffee shop, the facility's complex offered patios, pergolas, and quiet seating overlooking a small duck pond. Some amenities were beyond my mom's interest or activity level, but she could still enjoy the bistro, fireplaces, and library. We were emboldened when her hospice services were seamlessly transferred. Later, my mother told the assembled nurses and CNAs that she was content. A new hospice team met her in the common area while she was listening to the piano. (As time went on, that setting and activity would become her most comforting.) My small dog sat on her lap. The team noted that she greeted them with a smile, said she was looking forward to working with them, and denied any pain or immediate needs. Her "recent stroke" and the move "took a lot out of me," she reportedly said. (In truth, the disabling stroke, which she continued to describe as her "minor stroke," had occurred two and a half years earlier.)

A plaque at the entrance told a familiar story: a promise to create a comfortable home for elderly people and to improve upon the quality of care that had been received by a beloved relative. I'd read or heard about similar pledges in suburban Boston, in the state of Oregon, and in Wisconsin: Families frustrated by unhappy experiences embark on new facilities and innovative care programs for *others'* loved ones, who might soon be suffering from chronic diseases and dementia.

Although good intentions may be pledged, senior housing remains a *business*—a classification of real estate. Residents' private rooms, dining areas, and common spaces are planned and designed to utilize construction time and materials efficiently enough to maximize revenue per square foot. As in the hospitality and multifamily housing sectors, the income calculus works only if residents' rooms are *occupied*. A retired physician, an observant resident in my mom's first assisted living environment, had decided that the director was only interested in showing rooms to potential occupants. He said, "He's a real estate agent."

Within four months of my mom's arrival at her third facility, an exodus of staff members began. Five nurses left (three within one week), the manager of the secure memory care section submitted her notice, and the executive director either resigned or was fired (present on Friday, gone by the following Monday). During one tumultuous year, the director's position rotated among four different individuals—with four different leadership styles.

Caregivers transferred to other facilities or joined itinerant staffing agencies (some said good-bye, some simply failed to appear for their assigned hours, and a few walked away mid-shift). The activities staff, whose members had cared for my mom more consistently than the certified caregivers, became decimated. Almost every member left—except one talented and overworked music specialist—our favorite.

The specific, stimulating programming that I thought might occur in memory care never materialized. Colorful exercise equipment remained on open shelves or behind closed cabinet doors. "Want to see a movie?" became one long word: "Wannaseeamovie?"

As residents either moved to other assisted living facilities or died, vacant bedrooms were secured, and the staff removed telltale empty tables and chairs from the dining room.

Possibly because my mom was older, we were more affected by the turnover of personnel than we had been at her previous homes. She became disoriented and sullen as an ever-changing mix of temporary caregivers was hired from staffing agencies. Lacking on-site experience, agency caregivers tended to be distant, disengaged, and unfamiliar with the facility's schedule and the residents' needs. Some worked irregular hours, while others served for a week or two. Frequently, the temporary agency personnel outnumbered the facility's own employees.

Longer-term caregivers were sources of more consistent care, concern, and affection, but they struggled under constantly changing schedules, reassignments within the facility, and inconsistent supervision.

Evening attention was delayed by the prevalence of sundowning, the state of confusion that occurs in late afternoon and lasts into evening for people suffering from Alzheimer's disease and other dementias. Disoriented residents argued, screamed, and fought with their caregivers in the hours after daylight. When the need was greatest, the staffing level was lowest.

My aging mom had become a *two-person transfer,* and no one expected or wanted me to continue transferring her to bed by myself. Many nights, I paced while we waited for assistance. My mother dozed in her wheelchair, but she wanted to be in bed—and I wanted to go home.

To make matters worse, the dangerously inadequate number of caregivers was nearly always reduced by one CNA, because a difficult resident locked her door each night and demanded that one nursing assistant remain hostage until she was ready to release her—and she owned a cell phone (the only resident who had one), which she used at will to call the local police.

While caregiver attention was focused elsewhere, I sat with my mother, who awaited washing, toileting, changing, and evening meds, plus a transfer into bed. When she was still at her second place, I'd purchased a medically approved tubular bed bar from a medical-supply site. My mother knew how to hold on to the curved tube so that she could complete the transfer from her wheelchair to her bed. Although she was physically incapable of dislodging the bed bar, we anchored it under her mattress, according to printed instructions and warnings.

Every change in facility leadership produced challenges, and one new director demanded we remove the bar, claiming it was an illegal restraint. I reinstalled it several times, because I needed help when no caregivers were available, but the director appeared—unannounced—and quietly removed it.

When the nighttime wait became unbearable, I performed the bedtime routine without help and slipped out through an unalarmed side door, because I simply wanted to go home. My mother weighed less than 107 pounds, but her body was inert, and my right shoulder ached so intensely from the effort that I was pre-scribed exercises and PT treatments for several years after she died.

Acknowledging that the dearth of experienced staff was dis-ruptive and unsafe for my mom, the hospice agency scheduled two dedicated caregivers to assist with bedtime tasks on Wednesday and Friday evenings. We were still paying a premium rate for memory-level care, but the Medicare-reimbursed addition of hos-pice CNAs granted us respite, confidence, and occasional laughter.

On nights without hospice assistance, we were subject to the availability of either the staff CNAs, who were well-intentioned but overscheduled, or staffing agency personnel, who were sadly unfa-miliar with the facility's routine. I'm not a licensed medical pro-fessional, and I didn't have access to my mother's medications, but many evenings, I explained drug administration to itinerant licensed caregivers—the temporary evening med passers (medication aides).

I relaxed only when I knew my mom was finally cuddled under her blankets. Whether she read one article or even one word of one headline, I placed the day's *New York Times* in her hands, kissed her, and left. Frequently, I called a friend or my daughter-in-law in Denver to remain on the phone and monitor my lonely drive back home.

● ● ●

I continued to worry about my mother's care, and still wanted to help, but most mornings when I arrived and asked how she was, I witnessed the same confusion I'd seen at her previous residence. I was somehow in the way, or I was asking the wrong questions of the wrong people.

Not infrequently, caregivers from temporary staffing agencies didn't even recognize my mom's name. Simply seeking information about care and condition led to surprised and thinly veiled annoyance. *Advocate* is both a noun and a verb and, sadly, neither was appreciated.

Late one morning in August 2016, I received a call from one of the facility's nurses. She said she'd been informed of a "strawberry lump" on my mother's forearm but that my mom was not in pain.

I arrived while my mother was sitting in her usual lunch seat at a corner table—from which perch she could observe all the activity in the dining area—wearing the pale green outfit and hair bow we'd selected the night before. The allegedly painless lump had transformed into an ugly black-and-blue bruise, stretching from her wrist to her elbow.

I waited for someone to explain what had happened, and finally my mother looked into my eyes and said that someone had grabbed her, twisted her arm, and whispered, "I'll give you something to scream about." Sickened and so sad that I can still feel the loathing, I held up my phone and asked my mother to repeat what she'd told me, while I created a video clip. As moments slowly passed, my mother pointed to the offending caregiver.

When the bruise darkened and spread farther up my mother's thin arm, I decided to call the local police department. My mom had been physically abused.

Not considering it an emergency, a police officer arrived close to suppertime. Then, because she said she didn't want to cause trouble, my clever mom became an unreliable witness: She began to tell the policeman a story that started with her book club meeting the evening before! My mother was ninety-eight years old and had not participated in a book club for decades.

The police officer either didn't or couldn't insist on examining the bruised arm, and the events had exhausted both my mom and me. He ignored the pictures of the wound. He said good-bye, and he left. The assisted living nurse reported that I said, "the police officer determined no foul play," and the hospice notes repeated that there was no evidence of a crime. That became the determination, and nothing else was added.

I am not an attorney or a police officer, but I believe I understand the concept of hearsay. The determination that no abuse occurred relied on poor communication, unofficial secondhand information, and complete disregard of evidence. When I helped my mother undress for bed, I saw the clear imprint of fingertips— also turning blue—on her upper arm, above the bruise we'd reported earlier in the day.

The next morning, when I confronted the director, fully prepared to reveal who my mother said had hurt her, he turned to me and said, "You were the one who put her to bed." He was accusing *me* of hurting my own parent. I was too confused to react and didn't try to respond—and there was no witness to our conversation.

In the evening, two caregivers came to my mom's room to say they'd heard about the director's accusation. They'd helped my mother to the toilet during the night before the incident, and said they knew she was not bruised or injured when they assisted her; otherwise, they'd have filed a report.

At my urging, the hospice nurse and visiting hospice doctor (who would appear at various times during my mom's remaining days) met with us after the strawberry lump produced a hard ball of matter under the skin of my mother's forearm. The lesion wasn't painful, but it remained puzzling and required a long while to dissolve.

I remember being aware that the visit was out of character for a hospice team. They weren't certain where to meet and finally arranged three chairs (plus my mom's wheelchair) at the side of the TV-watching area, while remaining ever so careful to stay out of earshot of the residents who were watching TV. They had HIPAA privacy regulations on their minds but did not provide a diagnosis or any advice concerning my mom's arm.

Four days later, we attended an extraordinary care conference that included the director of the facility and one of his supervisors from the corporate home office. My daughter, who was director of crime victim services in the state's attorney general's office, joined the meeting and appeared with her official clipboard clearly visible. She led the discussion.

We never accused the caregiver my mom had pointed out, but we were told she was on suspension. We responded that we didn't want her to work with my mother again. We heard that a report would be made to the state, and my daughter requested a copy of the account that the facility would send to the state once their investigation was completed.

I never saw a report.

A hospice nurse noted that my mother was "unable to tolerate pain" and that she reacted to light touch on her sore left arm.

Although I had pictures, no one reviewed them. Even the clerk at the shop, where I had copies made, turned away from the shocking wound images. No one at the assisted living facility or hospice agency documented or discussed the telltale blue finger marks on the upper arm.

Assuming that it was a protected personnel matter, I heard nothing else—similar to the unwanted sexual advance at the previous residence. The next summer, in a casual conversation about CNAs moving between facilities, the former director of a different assisted living residence told me that the caregiver my mother identified had injured a resident at another location in the same city and had been fired.

• • •

Our worst days were still ahead. On September 1, 2016, I received the first hint of a baffling and ultimately fatal condition: My mom was observed to have had a "small nemesis," which the facility nurse thought might be due to a swallowing issue. This was sudden and strange. Not knowing how to proceed, I asked for several hospice visits—my fallback response.

By mid-September, my mother displayed "increased behaviors, hitting, biting, pulling at her hair." The hospice physician was making adjustments in antianxiety medications, and the frequency of falls (both witnessed and unwitnessed) was escalating. But, most serious—in retrospect—was my mother's "new and worsening cough with wheezes."

Within nine months, her notes read, "frequent coughing episodes with large amounts of clear sputum production." We were being distracted by behavior aberrations and escalating falls while unknowingly witnessing a slow death by cough.

Meanwhile, in her attempts to reach the toilet during the night, my mom continued to slip out of her bed, scooting or crawling toward the bathroom toilet. Once or twice a month, I was awakened by the voice of a remote corporate nurse—three hundred miles away—reporting a fall. Unwittingly, we'd stumbled into a multistate assisted living organization with structural weaknesses in communication—the precise area where we needed strength. My mom required more personalized attention than a telenurse simultaneously monitoring and responding to overnight emergencies in multiple midwestern facilities.

Even the hospice team was disempowered by the third facility's telephone system: Nighttime calls were answered in the RCAC's independent living section, but my mother was sleeping in the memory care unit. The two areas were separated by a long hallway, which seemed as daunting to cross as a military-training obstacle course.

One night in June 2016, a CNA (following standard procedure) had alerted hospice that my mother had fallen. The call was made before 10:00 P.M. When a hospice nurse requested further information, the residence staff member who was answering phones responded that he worked "on the other side." Worse, he did not know which of two numbers reached the memory care section. Only at 4:00 P.M. the following day was the assigned hospice nurse fully apprised about the fall.

I began to fear that our goals of health and safety were not attainable, and my mom told me she was ready to leave. Armed with fresh resolve but little free time, I drove as far as I was comfortable and searched for the ideal assisted living space, as the state regulations intended: "a living environment for residents . . . as homelike as possible."

I had no direction, and I was reluctant to seek additional suggestions from friends and family. The state ombudsman knew all the facilites in the region, but she couldn't make a recommendation. (That does not mean I didn't ask her to do so.)

Then, the marketing director, a friend who sometimes appeared in colors and patterns to match my mom's outfits, told me she'd met a lively, knowledgable facility director in a town thirteen miles away. I made an appointment and drove east. The facility, a ubiquitous free-standing structure, was newly remodeled, clean, and neat. Two small rooms were available. Both had views of trees. Sitting at a high conference table, on a tall chair better suited for a bar, I made a date for the director to evaluate my mom and left a deposit check for assisted living residence number four.

The morning we began processing a transfer with the director of the fourth facility, the hospice team, and my mom's PCP, my mother started to become less responsive and to twitch all along her left side. She was suffering another ministroke. Her care notes reported that she was non-verbal, yet they observed, "She did grab a staff member and her daughter's hand and bring it to her mouth to kiss it." While comprehending our intention to move to another location, my mom showed us *how much* she was craving a more perfect environment. The director of the new facility seemed to have witnessed whatever she needed for acceptance, but we all knew we had to wait.

● ● ●

After a few weeks, I took my mother to see the new site. Since it was Sunday, the director wasn't present. My suspicious mom immediately objected to the atmosphere. She told me it was "a place where people go to die."

A family of four was sitting in front of a large TV, and two people were rolling back and forth in their wheelchairs. The caregiver on duty was the manager's nephew. I thought a family connection was probably a good thing, but I never saw him again. The only other assistant told me she'd been employed for two weeks and couldn't answer any questions. I never saw her again, either. My mom whined and argued with me during the drive back. She was unaware that I'd made a deposit, but after I heard her reaction, I asked to have it returned.

Over the winter and spring, I visited or drove by almost every other free-standing assisted living facility in the county. Most seemed to have been built in the late 1990s—during the nation's initial wave of assisted living construction. A few had received upgrades, and several had come under the ownership of national corporations. Over time, many had become dated, shabby, and surprisingly cluttered. My mom couldn't live with clutter. Neither could I. We both deserved a peaceful, secure, and orderly atmosphere.

At the end of May, I revisited the building that had made my mother uneasy. The grass was green, flowers were blooming, and a large corner room was empty and inviting. I saw no other option, and I started to make new plans for a risky relocation.

● ● ●

Throughout our assisted living journey, I held to the false hope that my mother would become a recipient of care at the hospice agency's inpatient complex, within twenty minutes of my home. I visited, brought a friend for a tour, and submitted registration forms. In the winter of 2016, I scheduled movers two different times, but I was dissuaded when I learned that the hospice facility was designed for bedridden end-of-life patients.

Undeterred and unconvinced, I continued to dream about my imaginary solution: My mom would receive round-the-clock observation, nutrition, and care within the hospice environment. She would be surrounded with flowers and art, and her bedroom would open to a garden patio. Other friends and acquaintances transferred terminally ill loved ones to hospice, and, although my mother was still capable of activities and socialization, I had difficulty accepting how premature it would be if she were admitted.

Living in denial and my own fantasies, I reached bottom during a spring afternoon towards the end of my mother's tenure at her third assisted living facility. While sharing a wheelchair stroll to the water-retention area/duck pond at the south end of the residence, I received a call from one of my sisters-in-care, whose mother had been a resident at the previous assisted living home while my mom was there.

My friend told me her mother had been at the hospice facility for several days. I didn't comprehend the nature of the call: Her mother was near the end of her life. In my mind, admission to a hospice residency represented the ultimate gift of care.

My mom knew I was absorbed by the phone call and began perseverating about one of her issues: "Where's the dog?" or "Did you eat yet?" Because I was misguided and intensely envious, I peppered my caller with questions.

When I couldn't hear the answers, I told my mother, "Shut your [expletive] pie hole." I'd never voiced those words before (well, maybe the expletive), and I have no idea where the phrase came from, except for the years of overhearing my three teenagers bicker and argue with one another or with their young friends.

One of the CNAs—eating her lunch in a parked car near the side door to the complex—overheard me. Within a half hour, I was sitting across a conference table from the executive director.

Contrite and ashamed, I said I regretted my outburst and admitted to both the director and to myself that I was not coping well. I asked to leave the meeting as quickly as possible, because I wanted to sit next to my mother and absorb her love. I hoped she hadn't heard me, but, obviously, the juvenile and hurtful words were clearly articulated.

In reflection, but not self-absolution, I now note how quickly the incident was reported to the director—while my mom's calls for help routinely remained unheard.

●   ●   ●

On the day my mother finally moved out of her third care residence, the friendly marketing director also left, further eroding the staff level. By then, almost a third of the rooms in the secure memory care unit were vacant. I cannot unsee the image of my frail mom waiting patiently, but knowingly, in her wheelchair while movers cleared out her room and loaded her belongings into the back of a truck.

June 7, 2017 to October 4, 2017

Fourth Facility

Clinging to my vision of what good caregiving for seniors should look like, my mother and I proceeded with one more change. I was playing the mother/toddler game: pretending, for her benefit, that everything would be fine. I told myself that the uncomfortable earlier visit to the fourth facility was an aberration, and I looked forward to a decrease in monthly costs plus a new, relaxed atmosphere in non-memory care at a recently renovated CBRF.

Several professionals, including the nursing staff at her geriatric clinic, had either stated or agreed that my mom didn't require secure memory care. Wandering was neither in her nature nor a common symptom of vascular dementia, and she couldn't manipulate her wheelchair to exit her room, let alone a building. The facility's manager also assured me the caregivers were long-term workers who were devoted to the company, and she didn't supplement her staff with temporary agency personnel. Yet, at dawn on her first morning, my mother was awakened and dressed by an employee from a temporary staffing service. I didn't have the strength to argue. I had to tell myself that what I considered reasonable expectations were simply not achievable.

● ● ●

As I write these words, a journalist, covering postpandemic commercial real estate, reports:

Specialized housing for older Americans has been around for decades. But shifting demographics are forcing the industry to diversify more rapidly across rates and services, yielding increasingly lavish residences for upper-income Americans as well as a growing number of affordable housing models.[12]

I wasn't expecting my mom to reside in lavish specialized housing, and she wasn't expecting amenities like a cinema room and a cocktail bar.[13] I wanted relief from constant worry, and I wanted trained caregivers to be present and available if something bad happened.

I expected that my mother would be clean, fed, and socialized—even in my absence. Now I was informed that after the move from the understaffed third facility, hospice would reduce twice-weekly bedtime assistance from two supplemental CNAs to just one helper—and my efforts would fill the gap.

• • •

We were in a different location but in a familiar care space. When I arrived in the morning, I met distracted assistants who'd either tended to my mom during the night or helped prepare her for breakfast. Now, seeking information about my own parent's condition led to silence, tactlessness, and (I suspected) criticism.

My mom was aware of the staff's attitude. In a spot-on description of ageism,[14] she said that the director fussed over and talked down to her, "as if she was telling stories to a child." But she said

---

12. Linda Baker, "Expanding Options for Senior Housing," *New York Times*, July 20, 2022.

13. Ibid.

14. "Dr. Robert N. Butler, a psychiatrist, gerontologist, and founding director of the National Institute on Aging, coined the term 'ageism' a half-century ago, describing the stereotyping of and discrimination against older adults." Paula Span, "How Ageism Can Take Years Off Seniors' Lives," *New York Times*, April 26, 2022.

that the director fussed over her only when I appeared; otherwise, she walked past her.

I sensed that the small staff took my questions as challenges to their competence. On my mom's second day, a pink felt flower appeared on her door—a gift or a found item from the director. Even today, I keep the flower in my bedroom as a reminder of the passive approach of one participant in my mother's long-term care.

• • •

A board near the entrance announced three or four daily activities,[15] but there was no staff to organize the listed events and little socialization beyond a weekly showing of four recycled DVDs delivered by volunteers from the public library.

Though there were quiet semiweekly bingo games, my mom had never enjoyed that pursuit and rarely participated. Either no one noticed that she had nothing to occupy her during those events or no one cared—so she waited for me.

Just as we'd negotiated wheelchair walks around three previous residences, we left for daily strolls through the surrounding residential neighborhood. My mom reminded me, as she always did, that I was her "whole life."

• • •

The company's nurse traveled between several remote facilities and appeared at my mother's fourth assisted living residence once every two weeks. While acknowledging that she herself was not a

---

15. The Summer Fun schedule for July 2017 included Noodle Fun, Table Trivia, Hangman, Movement to Music, Read WSJ (*Wisconsin State Journal*), Stretch Our Arms, Let's Listen to Accordion, Dog Days of Summer Spelling Bee, Let's Tell Jokes, Bugs Bunny Birthday, Evening Stroll, Chicken Soup, Nibble and Natter, and Ball Toss. To my knowledge, none occurred.

nurse, the director said she could handle most situations, because she'd been "in the business" for so long. During the evening (sundowning) hours, there was often no supervisor on-site, and I could hear screaming coming from other bedrooms. I knew the young CNAs were not only working hard but overworked, and I became reluctant to leave my mom—usually staying long after she was finally in bed.

When our summer birthdays approached, my daughter reestablished a tradition we'd held for many years but had neglected in the recent summers that had followed her grandmother's stroke: She made plans for the two of us to attend a nighttime performance of *A Flea in Her Ear,* by Georges Feydeau, at a nationally recognized summer theater, located about thirty miles away.

Excited to spend familiar mother-daughter time (after so much intense daughter-mother time), I agreed. But as the day approached, I became unreasonably fearful of being away from my mom. I worried that she was receiving little to no care—at a facility that was being paid to *provide* care. I was constantly on emotional alert, even though there was no impending emergency.

More than anything, my mom loved seeing me with my children. Knowing that my daughter had invited me would have been as beneficial to her as a dose of antianxiety meds. If she'd been aware of my distress, she'd have insisted I go, but I canceled the quintessential summer evening and met my daughter for a late supper instead. I've ruminated over and regretted my overwhelming, debilitating insecurity ever since.

• • •

When the company nurse finally made a visit, the director informed me that the nurse would not meet with or care for my mom, because she was receiving hospice care. That disconnect wasn't the case at any other facility. Previously, nurses had cooperated with both the hospice staff and my mom's PCP for medication and care adjustments.

On July 5, less than a month after I relocated my mom to the residence, the director handed me a letter from the owner saying we'd have to leave within thirty days. The letter alleged I wasn't happy and that I'd raised my voice.

I recalled the morning before when I realized that my mother hadn't had a shower in several days. Because the usual hospice CNA would have Independence Day off, I had agreed that the assisted living staff should administer my mom's shower, and the director had confirmed the plan. Yet when I'd visited for lunch on July 4, I'd found my mother sitting alone in front of a TV—neither showered nor bathed. I couldn't remember if or why I'd been annoyingly, threateningly, or inappropriately loud. Now any apology seemed meaningless.

The state's long-term care ombudsman responded that the format of the letter and the grounds for the dismissal were invalid. Reasons for involuntary dismissal are listed in the state's administrative code. (Neither happiness nor tone of voice of residents' family members is included.)

(b) *Reasons for involuntary discharge.* The CBRF may not involuntarily discharge a resident except for any of the following reasons:

1. Nonpayment of charges, following reasonable opportunity to pay.
2. Care is required that is beyond the CBRF's license classification.
3. Care is required that is inconsistent with the CBRF's program statement and beyond that which the CBRF is required to provide under the terms of the admission agreement and this chapter.
4. Medical care is required that the CBRF cannot provide.

5. There is imminent risk of serious harm to the health or safety of the resident, other residents or employees, as documented in the resident's record.[16]

One month was hardly sufficient to acclimate an old person—or her daughter—to a new care system. We'd barely unpacked, and I was working too hard to know if we were unhappy or not. My mother had become quiet and self-focused, but from what I had observed of her interactions with hospice personnel, she was calm and cooperative.

The day after I received the eviction notice, the hospice nurse observed that I was experiencing caregiver stress and encouraged me to take breaks for self-care. She recommended Al-Anon meetings and consultation with the Dementia Alliance. At last, someone seemed to detect my discomfort. I didn't resist, but what I really wanted was a referral to the elusive world of stability.

Fifteen days after the eviction, I received notice that the assisted living facility had informed the state that they were rescinding the discharge. Apparently, the concerns had been sorted out.

Being allowed to remain was a proverbial mixed blessing. Because my mother was still falling or rolling out of bed, the staff were working to adjust her sleep patterns. They'd suggested waking her up early—one of the first for breakfast—and trying to keep her up later at night. Gradually, she began to refuse to take her antianxiety medications or eat her meals. When she became angry with me, her sundowning became more pronounced. She seemed to snap at around 5:30 P.M., displaying evening and bedtime behaviors that were unpredictable and potentially dangerous. Because I wanted to remain until my mom was sleeping, I left exhausted—driving home with my dog late at night.

---

16. Wisconsin Administrative Code, Chapter DHS 83, "Community Based Residential Facilities," Subchapter V—"Admission, Retention and Discharge," DHS 83.31—"Discharge or transfer."

To reframe a social connection, I frequently lingered to chat with the woman across the hall. She was always watching the same sitcom and knew each segment by heart. She told me nightly that she was waiting to regain her strength so she could return to Florida, but I knew we were both living under the illusions we'd created to survive moment by moment—day by day.

• • •

As suggested, I began seeking advice and counseling from the National Alzheimer's Association, calling its 800 number to unload my concerns. I remember sharing the association representative's suggestion that we all back off and give my mother space when she became belligerent. The hospice nurse validated the intervention, and later reinforced the caution not to meet anxiety with anxiety.

Because my mother called for me when I wasn't with her, the often-discussed and well-intentioned concept of being present *less often* appeared counterproductive. Frequently, when I left for coffee or a visit to the nearby thrift shop that we'd plundered when my mom was still living independently, I received calls from staff members, asking me to return.

Still, the assisted living director had two versions of reality. Either her patient experienced agitation in the afternoons when I was not present, or her patient's anxiety was worsened by my presence throughout the day. I had one mother and only one focus. I hoped for calm days as much as the director did, and I tried to stay out of her way.

• • •

As soon as I found my mom sitting alone, staring out of a window in smelly adult pull-ups, I knew I had to spend more hours accompanying her, rather than fewer. Yes, the frustration-driven, abrupt motions, like swatting away help when she wanted to move out of her wheelchair, left me aching, even winded, but my mother greeted me with a smile and a kiss whenever she saw me. She giggled and asked, "How did you know I was here?" and she never told me to go home. She was my motherless mother; I was her helicopter daughter, and I'd made a commitment to see her through—to the best of my limited ability.

Feeding myself fast food or walking my tolerant dog felt over-indulgent, but, finally, when I located a nail salon within walking distance, I started making appointments for pedicures. I knew there was an Al-Anon clubhouse on my way home, and when my evening commute coincided with meetings, I walked in. I remained for the full hour and listened, but my acceptance had dissipated, and I was too self-absorbed to share or receive help.

*   *   *

In my heart, I knew my mother was bereft about her situation—sometimes incapable of communicating, except by lashing out at all of us. Nothing and no one could dissuade me from feeling responsible.

During a care discussion with the state's long-term care ombuds-man about the facility's statutory obligation to offer meal substi-tutes for residents' dietary needs, tastes, and religious preferences—for my Jewish mother, no pork, ham, or shrimp—I heard the owner say, "Well, you know, this is a Catholic community."

Although I had to hope the climate could change, I didn't want my mom to remain in a community that wasn't capable or prepared to embrace her. Once again, I started investigating care options.

Now I broadened my search to include skilled nursing facilities—which were not appropriate, considering my mother's stable physical condition. In one home after another, admissions personnel refused to accept her. Our problem wasn't my voice, my habitual presence, or my mom's aggression, but the fact that both her PCP and the hospice physician had prescribed behavior-modification medicines—eventually introducing the psychotropic drug Haldol.

We were trapped in a catch-22 paradox: To control dementia-induced agitation, my mom was ingesting prescribed medication, but because she was taking specific drugs, she was not welcome at any other long-term care residence. We were stuck, and I continued to temporize.

Trying to relieve the caregivers, I wheeled my mom outdoors during the pretty summer afternoons. The resident across the hall joined us as I read chapters from the recently published *Shattered*, a recounting of Hillary Clinton's 2016 presidential campaign. My mom knew how the story ended, but she listened and made comments, as if it were still possible for Hillary to win. We all relaxed as we lingered under the single leafy maple tree in front of the building. Unknowingly, I was steeling myself for an upcoming onslaught of debilitating events.

• • •

My mother was cycling down. Sunrise to sunset, she dozed in her wheelchair and was periodically observed by hospice visitors. Unless I was with her, my mom sat near a side window, close to a common TV. I often found her alone, embarrassed by wet or soiled underwear. "I asked for help, and they said they'd be right back," she'd say.

Although she wouldn't discuss it, I knew from her laundry that she often slept in a wet bed. She broke my heart when she repeatedly told me, "This is the worst place of all." By the time we left, my mom had met and socialized with only one or two of the nineteen other residents.

Even though state statutes, codes, and regulations intend that "care and services a resident needs are provided in a manner that protects the rights and dignity of the resident,"[17] my mother referred to the caregivers as "fake" and told me they were "insincere."

The hospice agency continued to send an additional CNA to help with bedtime on Wednesday and Friday evenings, but we knew she wasn't receiving the basic care or attention she deserved. Because my mother fell asleep early, the assisted living director had adjusted the timing of Tylenol doses, but additional changes to medicines remained beyond her legal and ethical purview. For several years, family members had warned me, "Don't let them prescribe antianxiety meds." I was aware that the hospice physician had conferred with my mother's PCP to discuss antianxiety drugs, but I'd become less capable of understanding or monitoring medications, and my mom was nearing the twilight zone of chemical symptoms management.

One summer afternoon while I was out of the building, a facility CNA gave my mother an "as needed" Haldol dose. She told me my mother kept trying to get out of her wheelchair and would not settle down, even with distraction. Daily Haldol had been added to her schedule of drugs on July 18. I read that it was a powerful antipsychotic prescribed for managing schizophrenia.

On July 24, I asked a hospice nurse about as-needed use of antianxiety medications—both lorazepam, which was administered to control her seizures, and Haldol. The nurse confirmed that both drugs were delivered on schedule, and neither was intended for dosing without conferring with hospice.

Two days after, I met with the hospice physician to discuss my mother's medication regimen. He suggested adding an antihistamine, which could be calming, especially in elderly patients

17. Wisconsin Administrative Code, Chapter DHS 83, "Community-Based Residential Facilities," Subchapter I—"General Provisions,", DHS 83.01—"Authority and purpose."

with recurrent agitation related to dementia and aging. To monitor effectiveness, we should only make one medication change at a time, he said. Neither his words nor approach indicated that my mother was currently stabilized or would stabilize in the next six months.

I knew the nonmedical assisted living facility's director disagreed about whether she needed to ask her staff to contact hospice before administering supplemental Haldol. All I could do was remain present, try to distract my mom, place my dog on her lap, and take them for walks outside of the building. I trusted that the universe would somehow take care of us.

Given my lack of medical training and pharmaceutical experience—and my need to remain sane—I tried to forget about Haldol and focus on medicines for my mother's chronic cough. (One month before my mother died, Haldol was abruptly discontinued, and I couldn't interfere even when I read warnings against stopping or changing the daily dose.)

• • •

On September 20, as I was sharing my weekly coffee break with a friend—the hour when I allowed myself to be stress-free—I received a phone call from an unfamiliar social worker, who told me the hospice staff had somehow made the determination that my 99.5-year-old mother was not declining, and they could no longer predict a six-month life span.

The caller asked to meet with me that afternoon and said they were discontinuing care services in forty-eight hours. I took my mom and my coffee-hour friend (my second pair of ears) to the late-afternoon meeting in the sunroom adjacent to the assisted living dining area.

The social worker brought the hospice physician who had prescribed the antipsychotic chemicals that were preventing my mother from being accepted at other long-term care sites—the same doctor who'd appeared at the previous facility when I asked for help with my mom's bruised and injured left arm. "I need your help," I said to him. Once again, he was unmoved.

Insisting she had something to contribute, the facility's director invited herself to the meeting and told us that, without hospice assistance, my mom couldn't remain in the home. That condition had not been stated in our preadmission discussions, but within twenty-four hours, the manager gave me a second letter of dismissal, which she signed and CC'd to the president (and owner) of the assisted living facility and to the state's long-term care ombudsman (via email).

I was overcome with sickening bewilderment about my inability to sustain dignity and respect—at any cost—for my good mother. Standing in the small room that had become her world, I read, but couldn't process, comments about her "abusive" actions ("often biting, slapping, and yelling").

The letter alleged that the facility's staff had worked to tweak my mother's behavior medications, but, by their own design, I knew that no licensed nurse from their company had ever met or examined my mother.

Although hospice had determined that my mother's condition was *stable* and had discharged her, the owner of a CBRF licensed to serve residents of advanced age and/or irreversible dementia and/ or Alzheimer's wrote that, after only four months of residency, my mother's dementia had progressed too far for her to remain there.

The letter cited state code and the admission agreement I'd signed two and a half months before, when I was under duress and made the common error of family members: signing without considering the small-print implications.

• • •

My mother and I were involuntarily dismissed from her fourth facility. Almost five years later, an investigative reporter wrote that "national experts recommend that residents refuse to leave when told to do so, instead insisting on due process."[18] No one was more expert than I was on my mother's inability to withstand a legal battle. We were leaving.

I would have apologized or offered my regrets to anyone who was hurt, and, in time, I asked the head caregiver which staff members had been attacked or abused by my mother. Possibly because she was not allowed to discuss such things, she said she couldn't remember any incidents. Then she rolled up her sleeve and pointed to a location on her left forearm, implying that my mother had bruised it. I said, "I'm sorry." I really was.

In her eviction letter, the facility's manager included one suggestion for relocation: a secure (and presumably more costly) memory care building owned by the same company—located on a busy traffic corner next to a state highway. I demurred, although I'd only driven by the outside of the structure.

In a compassionate gesture, the manager mentioned a new facility at the southern edge of the county. She based her recommendation on one fact and one calculated assumption: "They are new; they probably have openings."

•   •   •

Wisconsin code outlines notice and discharge requirements for a discharge by a CBRF:

> 1. Before a CBRF involuntarily discharges a resident, the licensee shall give the resident or legal representative a 30-day written advance notice. The notice shall explain to the

---

18. Bill Lueders, "Evicting the Elderly: 'A Sad Thing That Happened,'" *The Progressive Magazine,* August 18, 2022.

resident or legal representative the need for and possible alternatives to the discharge. . . .

2. The CBRF shall provide assistance in relocating the resident and shall ensure that a living arrangement suitable to meet the needs of the resident is available before discharging the resident.[19]

Since she was no longer eligible for hospice care, I did not want my mother to remain as long as thirty days. I wasn't seeking any alternatives to the discharge, and I certainly did not want to transfer her to another facility owned by the same eldercare business.

During ten days of emotional upheaval approaching panic over the fear of running out of options (despite assurances from the state's long-term care ombudsman that my mom would not be "tossed on the street"), the facility's manager provided no assistance—except chatting with us on the sidewalk as the moving van was being loaded.

Either forgetting or avoiding submitting records to area skilled nursing and memory care facilities, the manager finally told me that records transfers were my responsibility. For the forty-eight hours that hospice was still involved, I asked them to send their version of my mother's files to several area long-term care sites.

• • •

When the owner of my mother's next assisted living facility came to evaluate my mom for admission, the lead caregiver said she had no computer access and couldn't make a copy of my mom's care plan. Standing between us and a functioning copy machine, she watched as we looked through the facility's only hard copy.

19. Wisconsin Administrative Code, Chapter DHS 83, "Community-Based Residential Facilities," Subchapter V—"Admission, Retention and Discharge," DHS 83.31—"Discharge or Transfer Initiated by CBRF, (a) *Notice and discharge requirements.*"

Going page by page, I took pictures of the document with my own iPhone.

Our only option was to move on. Three days later, my mother said farewell in the manner to which she'd become accustomed: Reportedly, she bit a caregiver in the arm.

October 4, 2017 to February 28, 2018

Fifth Facility

By the time my mother moved to her fifth assisted living facility, I'd almost earned a black belt in packing, unpacking, and introducing an elderly person to new surroundings.

Four years earlier, in September 2013, my mom was an inpatient in a stroke rehab unit. I'd selected a corner room in the familiar retirement complex that had become her world, and I registered her for assisted living.

A year and three months later, in December 2014, I'd helped my mother transfer to a more welcoming, orderly space. There, she became wheelchair-bound and spent fifteen months within increasingly confining walls. Eventually, it was clear that her needs surpassed the facility's capacity for care.

On a sleet-encrusted Sunday afternoon in March 2016, I'd visited a new residence that I'd heard about. The marketing director, whom I'd never met, and who hadn't been expecting my visit, welcomed me with warm food and affection. I hired a local moving company, began filling and labeling cardboard boxes with familiar belongings, and enrolled my my mother in a facility that included secure memory care. After a year and two months of organizational changes, remote management, and a dwindling staff, I moved my mom to a small suburban residence. I'd hoped to to simplify our lives, but before my mother could adjust to her new environment, we received an eviction letter. Four months later, we were officially discharged.

* * *

With my canine companion beside me, I drove thirty miles south. A young woman in hospital scrubs greeted me at the locked entry. "Hi, I'm the owner, and I'm a nurse," she said. I held my breath until she and her mentors decided if the fledgling franchise could accept my aging mom. The response was that they would welcome her *because* of her advanced age—so the staff could learn what was ahead for other residents. I sensed that a miracle had occurred. After four long years of searching for a different assisted living model, a caring family space had sprung up in the Midwest cornfields.

For almost a decade, while my mom lived in both an independent and assisted living residence a few blocks from my home, we'd been fortunate that the distance separating us could be traversed by a short walk or bike ride (for me). More recently, I'd been willing to drive twelve miles to nearby suburbs, but the location of this fifth facility seemed too far away—beyond my circle of comfort. My concerns were lonely rural roads in winter and the possibility of late-night emergency runs. I'd made two white-knuckle trips and one predawn trek in the past two years, and I didn't want to repeat those experiences.

Now, as my brave mother accepted one more move, I accepted a daily twenty-six-mile round-trip commute, and I began to reacquaint myself with the beauty of the golden autumn countryside. I never stopped worrying about my mother's care. I continued to offer help and hovered over her. When I arrived and asked how things were going, I had to be patient, but, in the spirit of cooperation and full disclosure, I was invited to review staff notes from the previous night and early morning.

Some of my mother's endearing traits reappeared: During the afternoon, she entertained herself and others by watching food preparation in the open kitchen; at night, she and I played her version of Bananagrams (as always, by her rules). She surprised the nurse/owner when she found appropriate letters for long words and spelled them correctly. She was still my clever mom, and "[l]iving in Dementia [wasn't] the defining chapter of her life."[20]

. . .

As my mother aged, she became obsessed with events in the news and common tasks. Still able to scan newspaper headlines, she remained reliable in recounting articles, such as those on local store and hotel openings.

One morning, my former advertising executive mom repeatedly told us about an attractive new coffee shop and restaurant—expecting that I'd take her there. A new lunch and coffee bar had been added to the upper level of the county airport. We had no plane tickets, but I wish we'd tried to visit.

She still recognized newsmakers (e.g., Donald Trump) on her TV and seemed to listen as I read chapters from *Fire and Fury: Inside the Trump White House*. Sometimes, I'd find her holding the book, staring at the president's angry face on the dust jacket.

Because she expected to pay for her meals, she began to obsess over dinner bills. I ordered a pack of cashier's checks, and we filled one out after each meal—the food, the charges, and the tip.

My mom knew when I was with her, and she loved my little dog, but she'd moved twice during the previous year, and she became disoriented—especially at night. Sometimes I read in the staff report that she'd tried to undress herself before rolling

---

20. Suzanne Finnamore, "Dementia Is Where My Mother Lives. It Is Not Who She Is," *New York Times*, May 11, 2022.

out of bed after midnight. I observed her routine only once, when she began to pull at her clothes and disrobe during a long day of uncooperative noncommunication—probably her final ministroke.

Thankfully, the facility's spirited atmosphere was conducive to a sense of well-being. The social woman who had spent a lifetime courting friends by sharing evenings or dinner out finally was acquainted with a dining area where she could linger and enjoy a variety of healthy meals—as attractive as I'd observed and shared when she was a resident of independent living.

My mom's diet expanded beyond that of assisted living dining rooms, where she'd relied on grilled cheese and tomato sandwiches. She was asking for second helpings, socializing when not napping, and smiling.

• • •

At 99.5 years of age, my mother might have thrived, but her cough and dementia were bringing her down. I persisted in trying to readmit her for hospice services. The same organization that, three years earlier, had been so eager to enroll my mom that it offered a contract twice, now continued to say she wasn't declining rapidly enough to be readmitted. A hospice team observed my mother sitting in the common room arranging pieces of a child's puzzle, and they told me her vocabulary was still too large.

On cold winter evenings, once my mother was in bed and before I headed home, I shopped at the closest Walgreens or Target to purchase bandages, cough medicine, incontinence supplies, skin creams, and mobility devices—the pricey items that had previously been supplied through hospice.

Towards the end of February 2018, my mom began to display extreme difficulty swallowing. Her cough was louder, now almost constant. After breakfast, I picked her up for an early morning appointment for a "swallow test" at the hospital. The CNAs noticed her food-stained shirt and tried to clean her as we were leaving the building—for the last time. In the end, the stains wouldn't matter.

· · ·

Six weeks before her one hundredth birthday, my mother was hospitalized with life-threatening episodes of coughing and aspiration pneumonia.

My daughter, who had helped move her grandmother from her Florida retirement home twelve years earlier, arrived to assist with a final relocation. Once again, we sorted, packed, donated, recycled, or discarded my mom's clothes, jewelry, books, pictures, furniture, linens, and accessibility aids. We took no furniture and very few items of clothing to her final assisted living home.

For her last month, my mom transferred to a higher, far more expensive level of senior care—her sixth long-term care residence—where she would receive one month of skilled nursing, until the announced relicensing and conversion of the skilled nursing facility to assisted living. Her suitability and acceptance, once questions for other facilities, were settled. She arrived by ambulance.

March 12 to April 12, 2018

Sixth Facility

In early 2006, my mother and I visited independent living apartments in a sprawling CCRC, but availability was limited, and she chose to live closer to my home. Twelve years later, on March 12, 2018, a private ambulance transferred a thin, sleeping passenger from the hospital to a sparingly furnished room in a new wing of that same complex.

Three weeks after my mom became a resident, the facility's state license classification as a health center (skilled nursing) changed to that of assisted living. Recalling a recent local newspaper account, I was vaguely familiar with the change:

> . . . converting its nursing home to an assisted living facility, a move that is relatively new in (the state) but could become a trend because of Medicare payment changes, authorities say. . . . The 44-bed nursing home, one of 19 nursing homes in [the county], will by April become a community-based residential facility, a type of assisted living . . . [21]

According to health reporter Wahlberg, critical differences exist between nursing homes and assisted living facilities:

> Nursing homes, staffed with licensed nurses and equipped to provide physical therapy and other medical services, are regulated by the federal government and inspected routinely by states.
>
> Assisted living facilities, which provide meals, housekeeping and assistance with personal care, have no federal oversight and varying degrees of state supervision. Staffing requirements aren't as strict, and staff typically have less training. [22]

The conversion trend had changed the face of the state's nursing home/assisted living industry in just nine years:

> Assisted living has grown rapidly . . . around the country in recent years, in part because many consumers prefer it to nursing homes. But regulators have expressed concerns, saying staff aren't always able to handle the increasing medical needs of assisted living residents.

---

21. David Wahlberg, "Converting Nursing Home to Assisted Living, a Possible Trend," *The Wisconsin State Journal*, October 30, 2017.
22. Ibid.

The state has nearly 4,200 assisted living facilities with a total of more than 59,000 beds, compared to about 400 nursing homes with roughly 33,000 beds. Until 2008, beds in nursing homes outnumbered those in assisted living.[23]

When I'd asked the hospital social worker about the implications of the conversion from skilled nursing to assisted living and the likely impact on my mom's care, I received a courtesy call from the facility's admissions assistant. She said, "Residents and their families prefer a more homelike atmosphere to that of skilled nursing."

The time had passed when I was asking to paint rooms, seeking a certain ambience. My singular goal was to help my mom receive dedicated and dignified end-of-life care. And so, we entered my mother's sixth and final assisted living location.

● ● ●

Theoretically, when she left the hospital, my mother retained the option of returning to her fifth residence, but her dietary needs were central to preventing death by aspiration. She could consume only thickened liquids, and all food had to be ground, mashed, or softened. The hospital dieticians had produced a steady stream of safe food offerings, and although state code requires that "[t]he CBRF shall provide a therapeutic diet as ordered by a resident's physician,"[24] I suspected that, even with their well-stocked kitchen and creative cooks, the fifth facility would be challenged, and I didn't have the energy to constantly oversee my mom's food choices.

23. David Wahlberg, "Converting Nursing Home to Assisted Living, a Possible Trend," *The Wisconsin State Journal*, October 30, 2017.

24. Wisconsin Administrative Code, Chapter DHS 83, "Community-Based Residential Facilities," Subchapter VII—"Resident Care and Services," DHS 83.41—"Food service, (2) Nutrition. (a) *Diets.* 2."

Thus, life-threatening coughing spells drove my mom's daily fee from $188 in a semirural franchised facility to $385 in a premier nonprofit institution—and the monthly rate doubled, from $5,625 to $11,550.

Swept into the dynamics of advancing age, declining health, dietary restrictions, and medical economics, costs became irrelevant. For my mother's last month, March 2018, I paid over seventeen thousand dollars in rent to *two* long-term care facilities (one, whose fee I'd paid at the beginning of the month, before she was hospitalized, and a second, where she was taken to die). My son said I should just pay, and I did. I had other issues to monitor.

• • •

On entering the skilled nursing unit, we attended a routine care conference. My daughter, who was still visiting, joined us in what turned out to be a mere twenty-minute roundtable of introductions to the nutritionist, activities person, and the facility's nurse/manager. We briefly discussed my mother's health history, including her previous assisted living facilities and her chewing and swallowing problems. The staff was also careful to ask about their need to be cautious "at times" due to the patient's history of biting. The remainder of the conversation involved ordering an oxygen mask, whether they could enable closed captioning for the common area TVs, and the timing of diarrhea medication. I'd looked forward to discussing my mother's diagnoses and needs—especially the required soft diet—but no one asked or listened.

I'd hoped to hear comforting assurances about dignity, comfort, and care. I wanted my daughter to learn that we were doing the best we could for her grandmother, our loved one. But the assigned hospice team failed to attend the meeting—even by phone, as they'd arranged—and my daughter's presence was not recorded.

I'd faltered through the lengthy path of my mother's physical decline, and I seemed to have relinquished my right to participate in meaningful care discussions. Every morning when I arrived and asked how things were going, the responses from staff members on her floor sounded scripted or dismissive: "I don't know. I just got here." Sometimes my mom's hearing aids were in place and functioning. Often, they were not. Sometimes her false teeth were in place, but she was resisting hands-on care, so most days they were not. After one CNA asked, "Is that important?" I began to perform my own ear and mouth checks. I reasoned we were being treated as short-timers, not as a family qualified to receive professional nursing services.

• • •

Every afternoon, as at all her assisted living residences, I wheeled my mother and my dog to a spot in front of a fireplace or a sunny window. In previous facilities, I'd discovered my mother by fireplaces and windows slumped in her chair, her head drooping towards her chest. I became determined to prevent the forlorn look that signaled care-facility neglect.

Physician and researcher Atul Gawande wrote, "As our time winds down, we all seek comfort in simple pleasures—companionship, everyday routines, the taste of good food, the warmth of sunlight on our faces."[25] Together, my mother and I had maintained her nightly routine of selecting an outfit for the morning—and looking forward to the next day. Because the task of dressing and undressing was made easier by elastic waists, I'd visited the closest Walmart and bought pairs of pull-up slacks in several colors. Many evenings, I found relief from the intensity of the assisted

---

25. Atul Gawande, *Being Mortal: Medicine and What Matters in the End* (New York: Henry Holt, 2014), p. 127.

living routine by lingering in Walmart on my way home, checking new colors on display—until my mother owned them all.

During her adult years, my mother had built her wardrobe from thrift shops and bargain basements, cultivating a stylish appearance. In assisted living, her style continued with colorful T-shirts and hoodies, hair bows, and sneakers. On happy days, she added Mardi Gras beads—and always lipstick and eye makeup. On her lowest days, following her recurring ministrokes, I knew she was improving when she smiled at us and asked, "Do I have lipstick on?"

While she could still sit in upholstered chairs in the small common living room at her second facility, I'd added a red-and-white blanket for her lap and placed her own footstool under her legs. Later, when wheelchair-bound, she developed an involuntary twitch and bruised the skin on her ankles and shins when they rubbed on the metal leg rests. With oversized needles and thick yarn from the nearby craft store, I knit bright pink covers to slip over the chair's sharper parts.

Now, in my mother's sixth facility, I still selected an outfit for the morning—but she no longer chose the colors. Then she no longer left her bed. A week before she died, I brought her three soft cotton nightgowns in pastel colors: pink, light blue, and turquoise.

● ● ●

My good mom died in a city that was my adopted home. When she was still independent but no longer capable of living alone, she migrated and became an active, recognizable member of a new community. Once she required assistance, she was shuttled between six private long-term care facilities—CBRFs licensed by the state. She was cared for, entertained, fed, appreciated, and loved; she was also hurt, bruised, neglected, marginalized, medicated, feared, ignored, and evicted.

I wish I could have provided more consistent care under more permanent conditions. I wish other models and practices had been available. Given our options and our willingness to pursue them, I still don't know how we could have selected an alternate route. Perhaps "Where [we] thought [we] were going to never was there."[26]

---

26. Flannery O'Connor, *Wise Blood* (New York: Farrar, Straus and Giroux, 2007), p.109.

Dinner Is Served

At any age, food and food service provide a sense of well-being, a pattern for the day, and a source of joy. Marketers are aware that dining room visits and quality guest meals can convince potential long-term care residents to move to their facilities. Wherever my mother and I searched for an independent living placement, we were offered lunches—sometimes with printed menus, and always with eye-to-eye attention from the serving staff. In contrast, assisted living visits—usually necessitated by health crises—are overshadowed by angst and need. Too frequently, decision makers overlook food considerations and seize opportunities to enroll loved ones as soon as spaces become available for occupancy.

In only one of my mother's six assisted living facilities was food preparation and service a holistic process—one that, from unpacking groceries to asking for seconds, my mother observed and shared. In five other locations, food preparation and quality approached unacceptable levels for her.

• • •

In my mother's house, the first question was always "Do you want something to eat?" Food was comfort, sustenance, and love. Soups came not from cans but from fresh cuts of beef and freshly soaked beans. Cookies and brownies (actually, date and nut bars rolled in confectioner's sugar) didn't come in packages—they were freshly baked. Within minutes, my mom could create a vegetable salad that included chunks of tuna and hard-boiled eggs.

Somehow, tea was always available. "Do you want a cup of tea?" she'd ask. Even when visitors came to her unpretentious and often crowded assisted living spaces, my mother insisted on offering tea. My job was to go to the kitchen area (sometimes locked) and retrieve hot water. My mom's responsibility was to keep a variety of tea bags in her room—and to offer warm drinks.

A common Jewish trope is "Eat, eat, we've got plenty" (even with the understanding that, at times, the promised bounty might be limited). Italian mamas are known to offer food to their children first: "Did you eat? Okay, I'll make you something." The love message is universal. The novelist Viet Thanh Nguyen said,

> . . . the way that Vietnamese express love is through . . . being concerned, on an everyday basis, with whether you've eaten or not. And this comes from being—you know, growing up in countries where food was a scarce resource and was a way of showing hospitality and love.[27]

After my mother's hip operation, my adult daughter sat at her bedside and gently fed her, and the nurse on the floor was reduced

---

27. "Race in America: History & Memory with Viet Thanh Nguyen," *Washington Post Live*. March 15, 2021.

to tears. When my son brought his family for what would be their last visit, we moved my mom away from the bland, unwelcoming dining area in her fourth residence to the sunroom (where we'd one day gather to be told that hospice was discontinuing service and we were being evicted). Without prompting or suggesting, my son picked up a spoon to feed his Nana Lil. This is what our elderly loved ones deserve.

● ● ●

At my mother's first assisted living facility, I had no reason to give any forethought to diet. The dining room in the independent living section received kudos from local food critics for "offering residents (and their guests) an opportunity to 'dine out' without leaving the building or coping with the vagaries of Wisconsin weather."[28] Not reported, however, was that a separate, utilitarian kitchen prepared lower-quality meals for the assisted living area, skilled nursing section, and employees' dining room. I had no idea that both the food product and service would convert from resident-oriented to institutional.

When my mom still resided in independent living, we'd shared lunches, dinners, and gourmet brunches. Everything was an excuse to eat out—before plays and the opera, after shopping, even after her haircuts. "I can't go home now. Everyone has to see this new style. Let's just have tea," she'd say.

Amazed and entertained, I watched my mother become a minor TV food commentator. One morning, she appeared in an interview with a local TV station about the recession of 2007–2009. I walked into her living room and saw her sitting in front of a camera, lights, and a mic, explaining—in her Boston accent—how

---

28. Nadine Goff, "Let's Eat: Seniors Dine with the Seasons," *Cap Times* (Madison, WI), May 5, 2019.

she'd stood in line during the Great Depression of the 1930s and bought only half loaves of bread (the first time I'd heard that story).

Another day, she portrayed a chatty senior receiving a bag of pricey groceries in a political campaign ad supporting a friend who was running for countywide office. "Oh, are these all for me?" my mom asked, looking and sounding like she'd been sent by central casting. The camera frame didn't reveal that she was so short that the actor, who presumably had brought her the brown bags loaded with food packages, was *kneeling* in the hallway outside her open apartment door.

With a ride back from the hospital on a stormy Thursday night, everything changed. During the next several weeks, while still clearing furniture and clothing from a comfortable apartment in the independent living section, I tried to adjust to the new rhythm of our lives. We would never again take our places at tables in the full-service restaurant on the lower level of a long-term care complex and share multicourse dinners with my mom's friends. Menus became posted charts—repetitive and often inaccurate, and staff attention to diet was diminished by both my mother's disabilities and the needs of those around her.

Over the next four and a half years, I learned the rules and procedures of institutional food service. I also monitored my mother's diet and requested or insisted on special foods—until the weeks when my children and I slowly and lovingly spoon-fed her.

· · ·

The Centers for Medicare & Medicaid Services (CMS) has developed protocols and guidelines on dietary management in *nursing homes*: "They shape the format and frequency of meal plans, pushing dietitians to craft suitable regimens that take into account all aspects of the resident's life —from their health to cultural preferences—to ensure each person receives optimal nourishment."[29] However, the CMS has little oversight of *assisted living*. It is up to residents and family members to make their preferences, needs, and voices heard. State regulations for diets and meals in Wisconsin's assisted living facilities are surprisingly few:

(2) Nutrition.

  (a) *Diets.*

    1. The CBRF shall provide each resident with palatable food that meets the recommended dietary allowance based on current dietary guidelines for Americans and any special dietary needs of each resident.

    2. The CBRF shall provide a therapeutic diet as ordered by a resident's physician.

  (b) *Meals.*

    1. The CBRF shall provide meals that are routinely served family or restaurant style, unless contraindicated in a resident's individual service plan or for short-term medical needs.

    2. The CBRF shall provide at least 3 meals a day, unless otherwise arranged according to the program statement or the resident's individual service plan. A nutritious snack shall be offered in the evening or more often as consistent with the resident's dietary needs.

    3. If a resident is away from the CBRF during the time a meal is served, the CBRF shall offer food to the resident on the resident's return.

  (c) *Menus.*

    1. The CBRF shall make reasonable adjustments to the menu for individual resident's food likes, habits, customs, conditions and appetites.

---

29. https://www.fooddocs.com/post/cms-dietary-regulations-for-nursing-homes

> 2. The CBRF shall prepare weekly written menus and shall make menus available to residents. Deviations from the planned menu shall be documented on the menu.[30]

Quite simply, assisted living facilities are required to offer palatable food, meet special dietary needs, and publish menus.

• • •

When she entered assisted living, my mom could still feed herself, but menus proved confusing. Even in her younger years, she'd been intimidated by food selections. Her Florida friends had noted—sometimes unkindly—that she mimicked their choices in local restaurants, and I came to suspect that during the long years of their marriage my dad had either gallantly or impatiently overseen her decisions.

In the past, when we settled into a restaurant, almost before opening our menus, my mother's first remark was, "Let's share something." Frequently, I'd order a dish I didn't want, because it was easier to cater to *her* preferences. I'd known for a while that she relied on a limited number of main dishes during her independent living years—usually salmon, another fish, or a hamburger. She chose food items as a Jewish woman who'd refrained from eating nonkosher offerings her entire life: no bacon, other pork products, or shellfish.

My mother's first assisted living facility menu offered two choices for every supper. The serving staff peered into food containers that were brought in insulated carts from a central kitchen and polled each resident by asking, "Pork or chicken?" or "Pasta or chicken and rice?" They offered an assortment of three small salads—yesterday's leftover salad plus two fresh

---

30. Wisconsin Administrative Code, Chapter DHS 83, "Community-Based Residential Facilities," Subchapter I—"General Provisions," DHS 83.41—"Food service."

ones. Dessert was frequently ice cream and store-bought cookies. My mother loved all ice cream, especially vanilla, and refused most of the cookies. While meeting state guidelines, the menu choices rotated through a set schedule and quickly became boring. I was surprised when dishes appeared that I thought were too heavy or spicy for aging digestive systems, and my mom assiduously avoided them.

My mom was free to choose her seat but gravitated to her usual place at a table for four, where she could watch over the dining room activity—sadly aware that she was no longer socializing with her circle of friends from independent living and no longer enjoying the dining experience she'd known.

As food names became unfamiliar or confusing, my mother became less willing to participate—quietly acting as though she didn't understand what the servers were saying. Predictably, she began to imitate Lois, a table mate whose favorite sandwich was grilled cheese and tomato on white bread—a comforting food combination that was tasty, familiar, and relatively easy for old people to order and handle.

Before long, additional residents wanted to be like Lois. Because there was no griddle or grill in the dining room, each sandwich was prepared in a single frying pan on the stovetop, creating an annoying time lag—a Lois sandwich supply-chain backup. More than a few residents requested and ate sandwiches twice a day, and I became aware my mother was habitually ordering grilled cheese and tomato—for both lunch and supper.

At the time, the monthly rate (rent, including food, activities, and care) at the assisted living facility was between five and six thousand dollars, depending on a resident's degree of acuity. One day, betting on both inflation and declining health, I looked at my mom and exclaimed, "That's a seven-thousand-dollar grilled cheese sandwich!" Indeed, as time passed, a ten-thousand-dollar grilled cheese sandwich became a more accurate estimate.

A Lois sandwich may have afforded a palatable meal that met state dietary guidelines, but besides the questionable nutritional value of a limited diet, the plain bread and cheese combination priced out to an inexpensive alternative that benefited the house. We were undoubtedly paying more for a lower-quality diet. My mom missed the salads, entrées, and desserts she'd become used to in independent living. When she was willing to accept canned soup, she balked at the only choices—low-sodium Campbell's chicken noodle or tomato—and told me they were tasteless.

Weekend meals were especially unappetizing. I told the director of the long-term care complex that serving a "football Saturday" meal of hot dogs and brats was not healthy for old people, and he told me that at their age, the ingredients made no difference.

Soon, my mother and I started frequenting the café in the independent living section. Although we effectively paid twice for my mom's meal (a daily lunch was included in the monthly assisted living invoice), additional incidental food charges no longer mattered. I was simply trying to buy smiles. I grew tired of asking the kitchen staff and facility directors to find other solutions and finally asked them to limit my mom's intake to *one grilled cheese and tomato sandwich per day.*

• • •

Not all assisted living dining rooms are alike. When my mother moved to her second residence, she was shown to a permanent seat—carefully selected by the head nurse—at a table for four, with carefully folded deep red napkins. Although there was a modern kitchen adjacent to the dining area, food was prepared in the facility's basement, delivered by elevator, and kept warm over large containers of hot water.

The knobs on the front of the oversized gas stove—plainly visible from the dining area—had been removed, presumably to prevent residents from accidentally turning on the burners. If my mother requested a substitute because of either unfamiliar food or religious preference, her wait was extended by the basement preparation and inefficient delivery.

Further complicating our lives, my mom was starting to show evidence of dementia sundowning by growing impatient, annoyed, and even hostile in the late afternoon and early evening—right at suppertime.

As required by the state, the director prepared weekly menus and was diligent in discussing meal choices with us. Substitutes for pork or ham usually appeared as either tuna fish salad or grilled cheese sandwiches.

My mom, frequently hungry, remained interested in meals, but she was starting to struggle with spoons and forks. Without intending to disturb the meal routine, I realized it was less complicated and more rewarding to bring a bagel and cream cheese from either a restaurant or my own kitchen and watch my mom grasp and eat familiar finger food, with a smile.

One benefit of the location was proximity to sandwiches from a Subway shop and containers of chicken noodle soup from a nearby Panera. I didn't have to be told that my mother wasn't the only hungry person in the dining area—there were others with special needs, including an entire second floor of memory care residents. Rather than fuss or wait for substitute dishes that she might not want to eat, I could leave the building and return with a meal in less time than it took for my mom to receive a special plate from the basement kitchen. If I attempted to analyze our food expenses, the daily price of her meals escalated every time I purchased an outside sandwich, but I began to look forward to the food missions— and the respite.

• • •

As with many residents of assisted living, the sphere of my mother's life began to shrink. Still, I managed to take her on short trips for coffee. When she became less mobile and transferring in and out of my car became difficult for me to accomplish by myself, a coffee date meant a drive to Dunkin' Donuts—just around the corner—and coffee in the car. We called our short rides "adventures."

During the year and three months when my mom was a resident in her second facility, the basement kitchen activity was disrupted by so many flooding episodes and recurring plumbing or electrical stoppages that the quality and palatability of the food output declined. While complying with the state's requirement for three meals a day in an assisted living facility, an increasingly large mass of prepared food was untouched and discarded—meal after disappointing meal.

My mother started losing weight. Once she became a recipient of hospice services, I asked her caregiving team to meet with the facility's nurse about the quality of food and dietary choices. Although the resident nurse was also the assistant director, she refused to collaborate because, as she said, she was reluctant to cross professional boundaries by discussing food with the hospice team.

One evening, while shopping at Target for pillows and a blanket to cushion a rigid wheelchair, I lingered in the housewares aisle and noticed panini makers tucked into the display of small kitchen appliances. My mom's room included an under-the-counter refrigerator that had remained empty—so now I stocked it with tomatoes, cheese slices, and white bread. With the impulse purchase of a small grill, I became our own chef. When things weren't working well in the dining room, I could cook and serve Lois sandwiches!

Too soon, I discovered moldy bread slices, green cheese, and unappetizing soft tomatoes—and I admitted that the functionality of the small fridge was limited. Also, I proved to be time-challenged as a short-order cook. Caught between preheating the appliance and monitoring the sandwich-making process in her bedroom, while explaining to my mother where I was going or where her meal was, I repeatedly either burned or undercooked the simple offering.

When I'd cleaned out my mom's kitchen cabinet in independent living, I'd found two shelves stocked with soup ingredients. Now, no longer the cook, she became visibly, almost childishly, excited when she heard or read that soup was being served in her assisted living dining room. But fresh soup that cooled off in the basement kitchen quickly lost flavor, became too thick to pour, and turned into an oversalted mystery serving. My mother's disappointment fed my growing sadness.

During one less than satisfying supper, I brought the facility's head nurse a cup of something my mother expected to be soup but was only a dark red mixture cooled to room temperature. The nurse didn't react, except to ask me to stop cooking grilled cheese sandwiches. Through her open office door, she had watched me go back and forth making sandwiches. As if I were her employee, she told me, "Oh, Judy! We don't want you to do this. You don't have to do this." But really, I did. My intention was to meet my mom's limited expectations about food and diet.

On a dreary spring Sunday, I left my mom napping and drove twenty-five miles to a suburban facility, where the marketing director offered me two soup choices: chicken and wild rice or tomato. I chose *both,* and within a week, we were planning my mom's move to her third facility, which had a large, accessible kitchen and consistent food availability.

Indicative of industry-wide employment dissatisfaction, and representative of problems that no family member anticipates on entering a care facility, the new head chef quit after three months, returned a few months later, then quit again. The assistant chef followed suit.

• • •

After my mom moved to her fourth facility, I realized that the cabinets in the large, open kitchen were sparsely stocked, and the meals were bland and disappointing. Even though the implicitly biased owner told me that my mother was living in a Catholic community, I continued asking for and expecting substitutes for the frequently served *unkosher* bacon, ham, and pork meals.

Most of the young kitchen staff could make grilled cheese sandwiches, and my mom ate them all—until one staff person told me it was odd to cook a tomato in the sandwich and refused to try.

The evening when the cook served each resident only one half of an egg salad sandwich on thin white bread and a half cup of Jell-O for supper, I was relieved and ready to accept the facility's unsolicited invitation to leave.

• • •

We reached the darkest moments of my mother's assisted living history—except for the days preceding her death—when she was evicted from her fourth facility and hospice dropped care coverage. My heart aching, I took her on a trip to order a new wheelchair.

As we were leaving the medical supply store, my mother told me she was hungry. By then, we'd been away from her facility for several hours, and it was past the posted lunch time. I asked the salespeople if I could borrow a sample chair to take my mom to the family restaurant on the other side of the large shopping area parking lot. "Of course," a kind voice said.

It had been so long since we'd eaten *out,* but now, during our most trying time, we were creating a precious food adventure. My smiling mom and I strolled toward the familiar chain restaurant, where we ordered grilled cheese sandwiches, soup, and vanilla ice cream. (We ate the ice cream first, before it melted.)

Although we didn't know it, my mother was savoring her last restaurant meal. She ate so eagerly that someone passing by told me it was a "beautiful thing" to see her happiness. I lingered and reflected on our good fortune—and relaxed.

• • •

I will always wish my mom could have lived at her fifth residence for a longer period. She was just starting to find her happy place—trying her hand at crafts, joining games of bingo, and playing word games with me in the evenings. When she could sit at the conveniently located counter and watch the activity in the open kitchen, she stopped calling for me.

The caregivers made regular trips to Walmart or Costco, returning with cartons filled with colorful packages of food and other supplies, and my mom loved watching the activity of unloading and storing.

Meals were varied and flavorful, and sometimes my mother ate two servings—of anything—pleasing everyone, but especially the owners and the cooks. I knew my mom was feeling cared for, and she was well fed.

Finally, my mother was in an assisted living facility with a functioning grill. Eating the first grilled cheese sandwich they created for her, she thanked the server over and over. I think I remember that she ate four during the next four days—because she wanted them, not because she couldn't or wouldn't eat anything else.

• • •

My mom's last Thanksgiving overflowed with autumn colors and textures—exactly how I remember the holiday dinners she cooked and served in our dining room as I was growing up.

The owners, for whom it was the first November in their new facility, made the day a family priority, rather than a chore for the caregivers who drew the shift. They arranged long tables, decorated the room in autumn colors, and circulated to make certain everyone was well fed. They personally thanked every family for attending.

I recalled two earlier facilities where I'd offered to help with holiday meals—happy to join in and relieve the caregivers. At my mother's final Thanksgiving banquet, I was a welcome guest amid an abundance of food. I wanted my mother to feel respected and special—well fed and celebrated—and I believe she did.

Refraining from unkosher foods was still confusing to the staff, and we had to be patient about substitute meals, but my mother was content in her surroundings. When the owner returned from a shopping trip with Hebrew National all-beef franks (which he said were the healthiest anyway), my mom exclaimed, "It's been so long since I've had one of these!" Indeed, it had been.

• • •

One January morning during her last winter, my mom fell from the toilet when the caregiver had walked away. She lost a tooth and sustained a laceration on her forehead. Her hospice coverage had been discontinued five months before, so the staff called an ambulance to convey her to a hospital emergency room. As I had done too many times, I followed the van.

The ER doctors determined my mother had sustained only a surface bruise. They didn't recommend any further diagnostics, and I agreed. During the typical extended wait for decisions, tests, and reports, I walked to the hospital cafeteria and came back with a grilled cheese and tomato sandwich. My mother was so happy with her meal that when she returned to her residence, she told the caregivers she'd eaten "the most delicious lunch at the Sears Tower dining room."

When the Sears Tower was built, it was the tallest building in the world—even taller than the World Trade Center's Twin

Towers. I knew the name had been changed to Willis Tower in 2009, but I didn't tell my mom. She was content with the memory of her celebrity lunch.

* * *

Of the fundamental offerings in assisted living (food, activities, and care), food should be the most sought after and treasured—the most carefully researched. But registration contracts offer no assurances that quality and quantity will be maintained. Beyond minimal state statutory requirements, nothing—not even a twice-daily seven-thousand-dollar Lois sandwich—is guaranteed.

One month after my mother visited her imaginary Sears Tower for lunch, she could receive no more grilled cheese sandwiches—just unpalatable softened foods and thickened liquids from a hospital kitchen and from her final assisted living home.

When my mom could no longer make herself understood, she smiled and fondled the folded cloth napkins in the sixth facility, where she was dying. I wanted her to feel cared for, comfortable, and well fed—but, beyond the dark blue napkins, I was helpless.

The last dining room was merely a place to eat. There were no conversations at the tables. Caregivers served prescribed meals, and sometimes, seemingly at random, they sat with or helped the residents. When someone thought to turn it on, a CD player added background music to the controlled confusion. I tried to remove my mother from the congested area as soon as she finished her meals, but I wasn't allowed to transfer her unless a caregiver accompanied us. While the staff was focused on other residents, we lingered in place.

Some friends met me to share lunches in nearby strip malls with surprisingly tasty offerings, but my food interest was elsewhere. My mother was wheeled into a dining room and then wheeled out. If we were lucky, she received nourishment. If we were slightly less lucky, she received perfunctory attention.

By early April 2018, there were no more folded napkins and no more sandwiches. After all the menus and reasonable requests, my mom lay in her bed—barely accepting the spoonfuls I offered. We'd run out of food adventures, and we waited.

Bait and Switch

As assisted living facilities have multiplied across the country, they've become increasingly competitive. Yet their radio, TV, direct mail, and social media messages all sound and look similar. These messages show smiling residents enjoying daily activities, birthday parties, and community get togethers. They assure us that all residents—especially memory-loss residents—are both mentally and physically active. Assisted living promotions are persuasive, and decision-makers like me can be seduced by a carefully crafted but false fear of missing out. The website of one nearby facility boasted a range of social accomodations, offering a social scene as well as time alone. At one point, I'd have said my mother preferred a social scene, but time and physical decline altered our outlook, and I learned the importance of pursuing our own options.

Like countless residents we met along the way, my mom protected her independence. She'd been an organizer, a top-level marketer and team leader at AT&T. Long before she was seated around activity tables in assisted living facilities, she was behind a desk—the beloved mentor to young women who worked with and loved her.

As a young housewife, my mother performed in community variety shows in our hometown—singing, dancing, and waving. She possessed an acute sense of comedic timing. She'd traveled through the New York Borscht Belt as a tourist, and somehow she'd acquired and perfected the art of delivering a joke: setup, story (often long), punch line (sometimes two). Even when she stumbled, her ethnic intonation and hand gestures were almost as funny as her jokes.

Within months of moving to her South Florida retirement community for residents over fifty-five, my mother became the president of the women's club. After my father died, she developed a stand-up comedy routine. She sent me programs from her volunteer performances, and only before her first talent show did she ever tell me she was nervous. After that, she was able to capture her audience—and she loved it.

As soon as she entered independent living, she approached the activities director with her typical eagerness to participate. She signed up for events in the common area: Halloween, birthday parties, and talent shows. With rehearsals, script revisions, and costume discussions, planning activities became her main activity. My mother coaxed her neighbors and friends to join the fun and convinced otherwise withdrawn retirees to participate. I became her willing wardrobe mistress.

We wandered through local secondhand clothing shops to retrieve essential costume pieces. I watched her climb creaky wooden stairs to excavate piles of old clothes on the upper floor of a resale shop intended for a college-age clientele. One day she told me to stand between her and the large street-level window, because she was disrobing to try on a white cocktail dress—right there. We bought a curly blond wig for her Marilyn Monroe appearance, and no one had to tell her what to do: She entered stage right, and without hesitation, assumed a husky voice to sing "Happy Birthday, Mr. President."

When a talented cabaret singer overheard my mom attracting an audience at an informal holiday gathering, she invited her to perform during intermission at a local piano bar. For the next several years, until her mid-nineties, we were Thursday-night regulars. Sometimes my mother just listened to the music, but on show nights, she fingered through her note cards, perched on a stool beside the piano, waited patiently for intermission, grabbed a mic and began by saying, "Now, quiet down, everyone!"

The startled bar crowd fell silent and waited for her surprisingly risqué jokes. My mom never failed to entertain; there was always one more story about aging people confronting their social and physical limitations. She selected her wardrobe for every performance: matching skirt and blouse, jacket, distinctive hat, and signature red or black pumps. Her brand of humor, decidedly Florida retirement by way of the Borscht Belt, attracted a following. She was a star.

●　●　●

Long before moving to congregate care, my mom lived in small houses overlooking the Atlantic Ocean. Although she and my dad held property on private beaches, she never learned to swim. Born decades before Title IX, she and her demographic cohort received scant training in athletic skills. The only sport I remember her playing in her adult years was golf—on the swampy nine-hole course in our New England town. But somehow, she learned the value of exercise and activity.

While still a resident of independent living, my mom had access to exercise classes, including swimming lessons. For the first time in her life, she swam, relying on foam devices to stay afloat. In the community workout room, she claimed a front-row chair, surrounded by a rainbow of colorful weights and training equipment. Sometimes I'd watch and listen to her count out the repetitions, "One, two, three," even when everyone else was quiet.

She stretched with pep and abandon. No one was surprised when she popped a muscle in her thin right arm, creating a permanent biceps bulge. Emergency room nurses said she was in good company; former Green Bay Packers quarterback Brett Favre had sustained the same injury. (Favre underwent surgery; my tough mom did not.)

My mom had always appeared physically strong, coordinated, and competitive. Although she would eventually become a needy senior, I trusted that she'd remain self-directed and engaged when she transitioned into an assisted living facility

• • •

When my mother was in the hospital recovering from her stroke, social workers visited to develop an exit plan. We knew little about what lay ahead, and we had no time to research the alternatives, which we didn't learn about until *later*. We were a target for brochures and social media posts about assisted living facilities that made my mom's future seem active and therapeutic. What would a resident or family desire more than the possibility of restored health and vitality?

Neither of us anticipated that my mother's active and purposeful lifestyle would suffer or cease to exist. After all, the messaging said daily activities were a priority. At each juncture, we had visions of fun—creating and maintaining community and regularly sharing adventures.

Once she entered assisted living, however, my mom stopped performing stand-up comedy. She retained her wit and sense of humor, but she couldn't keep track of her characteristically long stories. She also stopped swimming and taking exercise classes. Despite two rounds of physical therapy after her stroke, she never regained her core strength or sense of balance. She constantly rose from her chair or the toilet and stumbled forward, then ungracefully flopped into any chair she was facing. Updated mobility equipment helped, but nothing could restore her formerly independent lifestyle.

Expanding on the role I'd accepted seven years earlier, when I masterminded my mother's move north, I assumed even more responsibility as an advocate for the best-possible quality of assistance. I aimed to provide support as the consistent caregiver/daughter/only child/best friend of one good woman with poststroke vascular dementia.

Recently, I discussed this book with a slightly younger friend, who asked me what an assisted living resident would do without a nearby family member, loved one, or advocate. I had to admit I did not know. Sadly, the system is not designed for unaccompanied elders.

As my mother and I became a codependent duo, my days filled up with monitoring, reacting to, and overseeing new activities that I hoped would keep a nonagenarian with weakened cognitive abilities stimulated, occupied, and safe.

• • •

Assisted living media promotions, which boast a range of activities for residents, begin to sound like every day is play day and something is always happening. But my mother, oblivious to advertised activities, started lingering in bed. She watched CNN on her own TV, and she slept. I recalled a group discussion that was held during her week as a poststroke inpatient—how recovery might be enhanced by daily naps. I told myself my mom was healing.

After weeks of inactivity, one young caregiver surprised me when she said, "You know, all she does is sleep." I hadn't thought the dozing was strange or excessive, but I guess it was. I hadn't thought that my formerly engaging and energetic mother—Marilyn Monroe of a recent performance—should be entertained, but of course she should have been encouraged to remain active. That was the promise—the bait—in the advertisements.

Once her range of safe movement was constrained, my mother required and deserved a program tailored for seniors with diminishing abilities. I started to ask questions about—and participate in—her daily schedule, and I didn't stop until she died.

During one quiet after-lunch period, I'd noticed a phone number on a bulletin board for the state's long-term care ombudsman, and I made my first call to that office. The person who answered didn't seem to believe my description of my mom's sedentary existence. He'd asked when she'd last been out of bed for an activity. I'd hesitated, and then guessed it had been ten days. I wasn't sure if it had been that long, but I thought it had, and, as I spoke, I admitted to myself that my mother had been missing the life-enhancing assisted living amenities for which we were paying.

●   ●   ●

Similar to other states, Wisconsin has adopted code requiring daily activities in CBRFs, including in my mom's six assisted living sites:

> . . . to ensure all CBRFs provide a living environment for residents that is as homelike as possible and is the least restrictive of each resident's freedom; and that care and services a resident needs are provided in a manner that protects the rights and dignity of the resident and that encourage the resident to move toward functional independence in daily living or to maintain independent functioning to the highest possible extent.[31]

---

31. Wisconsin Administrative Code, Chapter DHS 83, "Community-Based Residential Facilities," Subchapter I—"General Provisions," DHS 83.01—"Authority and purpose" (2).

The regulations exist:

> Program services.
>
> > (1) Services. As appropriate, the CBRF shall teach residents the necessary skills to achieve and maintain the resident's highest level of functioning. In addition to the assessed needs . . . the CBRF shall provide or arrange services adequate to meet the needs of the residents in all of the following areas:
> >
> > > (a) *Personal care.* Personal care services shall be designed and provided to allow a resident to increase or maintain independence.
> > >
> > > (b) *Supervision.* The CBRF shall provide supervision appropriate to the resident's needs.
> > >
> > > (c) *Leisure time activities.* The CBRF shall provide a daily activity program to meet the interests and capabilities of the residents. Employees shall encourage and promote resident participation in the activity program. The CBRF shall develop and post the activity schedule in an area available to residents.
> > >
> > > (d) *Community activities.* The CBRF shall provide information and assistance to facilitate participation in personal and community activities. The CBRF shall develop, update and make available to all residents, monthly schedules and notices of community activities, including costs.
> > >
> > > (e) *Family and social contacts.* The CBRF shall encourage and assist residents in maintaining family and social contacts.
> > >
> > > (f) *Communication skills.* The CBRF shall provide services to meet the resident's communication needs.[32]

---

32. Wisconsin Administrative Code, Chapter DHS 83, "Community-Based Residential Facilities," Subchapter VII—"Resident Care and Services," DHS 83.38—"Program services."

Daily activities programs are prescribed by administrative code; regrettably, staffing issues, care requirements, and health crises intervene.

. . .

Those who devise advertising copy for assisted living facilities create impossible dreams, from smiles and stories to sitting outdoors in the sunshine.

Until her last weeks in assisted living, my witty, willful, competitive mom retained her desire to be social—and, if possible, the center of attention. When she was a resident of her fourth assisted living location, she said, "This is the worst place," she wasn't referring to health care, food, or safety; she was telling me she craved attention, socialization, and fun. My mother desired reassuring hugs, but who would provide them?

When she'd been healthy enough to perform comedy routines, my mom liked to mix long stories with short jokes that she called her "one-liners." She often included the joke about the doctor's nurse who says, "Doctor, there is an invisible man in your waiting room." The doctor responds, "Tell him I'm busy and I can't see him now." Unhappy in her institutional environment, my mom understood she'd become the invisible woman.

. . .

While health care institutions (skilled nursing homes, rehabilitation centers, and hospitals) employ both professional nursing staff and nonprofessional caregivers, assisted living and memory care facilities predominantly employ CNAs. The job descriptions are entry-level. Physically and emotionally handicapped residents might be waiting and hoping for one-on-one attention or engaging activities, but the CNAs are dispensing medications, toileting or dressing residents, preparing and serving meals, sorting laundry, making beds, or cleaning sinks and toilets. I observed overworked and undersupervised caregivers develop dispassionate attitudes and "It can wait" aloofness.

Unless designated employees are trained, equipped, and directed to organize games, exercises, crafts, music, and discussions, detailed activities schedules that are printed and posted on whiteboards are meaningless. Residents and their loved ones should not be misled by activities schedules that are displayed only because state regulators might drop in.

Shameless enticements directed to prospective residents and their families include impressive but insensitive notions. An advertising pitch might be addressed to former professionals (lawyers, doctors, or engineers) and suggest the facility would provide books and activities of interest. If someone loved art, music, or dancing, there would be specific programs for them, too.

In every activity room, we saw cabinets overflowing with puzzles and colorful exercise equipment (some, obsolete), but activities staff in only two of my mom's assisted living homes routinely unpacked the activity gear. In two residences, modern, presumably pricey computer software was on display and available to stimulate discussions, music, and memory games, but successful use depended on the training and creativity of patient, dedicated staff—and management support.

When the nurse at her second home showed us a large-screen computer, I was happy to open an email account for my then ninety-seven-year-old mother: grandnanalil@gmail.com. She was certain her messages came out of the back of the monitor, and I watched her turn the screen around after the first few times she hit SEND. Her biggest surprise was that we didn't place stamps on messages that she sent her great-grandchildren. "Ah," she said, "they'll think of a way to tax them." I replied, "Indeed they will."

One person at a time could access an exercise app and slowly stretch arms and legs, but that was not organized exercise, nor was it the strength-retention activity prescribed in my mother's hospice file.

. . .

Promises and posed Kodak moments belie the reality of ongoing monotony.

In six different environments, I observed no consistent, reliable path to regular mental, emotional, and physical stimulation. According to state code, activities must be held daily (with participation encouraged and schedules announced), but my mom experienced fully staffed, reliable programming only during her initial months at her third facility—and only until employee shortages contributed more to disruption and disappointment than to a healthy routine.

By the time she became a resident at her sixth and final congregate home, my mother was too weak to share—too exhausted to pretend to observe—planned activities. Volunteers distributed printed weekly programs to her room, and during a formal care meeting held during my mom's second week of residence, the activities director reported participation in a wide range of events. With my visiting daughter in attendance, and with her supervisors at the table, the activities director was not ashamed to claim my frail and silent mom had participated in a mobile petting zoo. By then, I no longer believed in the dream.

. . .

Carefully articulated lures hide the truth.

In four residences, my mom was parked next to disinterested companions in front of a large TV or near a sunny window—or both. At the third location, which attracted me for its experienced, engaging activities staff, my mom's attendance depended on her being wheeled to the activities area by busy CNAs. When they forgot or ignored her, she missed out. More than once, I found her flushed and sweating from hours of napping—forgotten and waiting next to a window overlooking an atrium, in the direct rays of the midday sun.

In two of my mom's more participatory environments, reading books and daily newspapers with residents was a popular activity, but on weekends, when managers were not present, the caregiving staff at two other facilities sat alone and read newspapers only to themselves.

My mother became silent and depressed when she sensed she was being overlooked. A simple game of balloon volleyball or genuine praise for choosing words for a group poem about the garden or the seasons would result in her sweet bedtime report. She'd say, "This was a good day." Sadly, those days were few and infrequent.

• • •

Assisted living advertising preys on the discomfort and guilt of absent relatives and loved ones. Carefully crafted wording makes programs and activities sound highly social, like substitutes for regular family visits.

Sometimes my mom was inconsolable and refused to attend events that bored her. Once or twice a week, a shower was her morning activity, and I accepted the fact that she'd be occupied and pampered for at least a half hour. If things went well and the caregivers understood her needs, she'd say, "I felt like a queen." If a new caregiver appeared and my mom had to explain her shampoo or hairstyle, she'd say, "That person had no idea what to do."

Caregivers who knew and loved my mom learned to distract her by applying cheek blush, lipstick, or eye shadow, and she responded with fashion-model–quality smiles. Foot care from visiting podiatrists provided professional attention, and manicures offered relaxed one-on-one time. More often than not, I was the manicurist, and my appreciative client held her relaxed fingers out, even if she fell asleep during the process.

I wasn't surprised when my stylish mother continued to wear a signature hair bow every day. She'd collected dozens of ribbons and owned enough for every mood, color combination, and holiday. Young caregivers at her second assisted living location asked to braid her hair and attach the bows, and staff in other homes continued the style. This pampering—unadvertised and personal—was priceless: We placed two large mirrors near the door to her room, low enough for viewing by a very short woman, and, eventually, by a short woman in a wheelchair. If I mentioned her braid, she'd say, "Oh, I never saw it," and I'd wheel her back in front of her mirrors or bring out a hand mirror so that she could admire, smile, and approve—for a second time.

If my mom was awake and cooperative, she'd participate in a group exercise—sometimes still remembering to count aloud—or she'd give a kickball a strong push that almost shot her out of her wheelchair. But when she was included in a daily circle facing a TV, my mother would tune out. "Please, I do not want to watch *Dr. Phil*," she'd say. Yet, day after day I'd find her immobilized in front of a TV with monotonous, unmonitored programming: soap operas, game shows—and *Dr. Phil*.

My mom would have left if she could have walked away. She would have wandered outdoors or into the solace of her own room, but she could no longer be trusted to be alone. My aging mom was trapped wherever she was placed, and I provided the only escape from the reality of her routine.

• • •

Promises of a healthy assisted living environment, camaraderie, and socialization don't magically materialize into a realm of well-being.

On our way out of my mom's fourth assisted living facility, as movers were clearing furniture and boxes from her room, I asked the lead caregiver why the staff wrote descriptions of three or four activities on the whiteboards in the hallways every morning. She probably knew my next comment would be "But you never prepare or present what you list," or maybe, "But you're not being truthful." She interrupted my thought. "Oh, that has nothing to do with us," she said. "It comes from our home office," and, with those revealing words, she walked out. So did we.

Only at her fifth residence did my mom trust that caregivers would respond to her raised hand or polite "Please, is there a ladies' room on this floor?" But, even there, she spent long hours napping beside other elderly residents on lounge chairs—all focused on random TV programming.

In that fifth assisted living home, we eventually realized my mother would prefer to sit in a wheelchair, bolstered by pillows, observing events occurring in the kitchen—from unpacking groceries to preparing meals. Alert for ever shorter time spans, she could be entertained by watching the busy staff. When she started calling it *her* corner, I realized the wheelchair-bound former comic had discovered a new, smaller stage.

• • •

On the spring afternoon when I write these pages, five years after my mother died, I receive a large glossy postcard advertising private tours at a new assisted living facility near my home: *Opening soon!* A full-color four-and-a-half-by-six-inch photo depicts two gray-haired people sitting together on the grass—blowing bubbles! In the background is a ten-speed bike handle with an attached bell and straw basket. My mother, who spent her professional career as a marketing executive for a national corporation, would have seen through the promises and hype. She'd have said the piece was "dishonest."

Assisted living is too complex to fit into a bicycle basket, and fluids are more likely to be urine, vomit, or thickened drinking water than pink bubbles. Marketing pieces should be required to be both truthful and helpful for individuals and families who are fraught with concern.

For my mother and her coresidents, assisted living offered beds, showers, and the expectation that state requirements would be followed in specific areas: meals, age-appropriate activities, and a limited amount of nursing attention, including dispensing of meds. To suggest that families and loved ones made life-changing decisions based on the opportunity to blow bubbles is insultingly ageist.

Bait and switch is considered fraud in retail sales; advertising that services and an active lifestyle will be present in the assisted living milieu, without intention or ability to provide them, must be held to the same degree of culpability.

• • •

Assisted living/memory care activities programs vary according to staff interest and training, budget, and residents' capabilities. What engages one resident might not interest many others. What engages one resident on a Monday or Tuesday might not prove entertaining for the rest of the week—or month.

One of the first observations I made was the problem of gathering all assisted living residents on my mom's floor to take them to a planned activity or event. Some people were napping, some needed encouragement, and many required toileting. More than once, an activity was scrapped because the first few residents lost interest and wandered away or fell asleep in their seats or wheelchairs, while others were still being rounded up. Timing was everything. Sometimes, a regularly scheduled activity plan worked out; other times, an impromptu gathering was more successful.

The activities director at my mom's first poststroke assisted living residence told me she invited residents to join in activities, like crafts or exercises, but she only asked twice. If anyone was sleeping, feigning sleep, or otherwise reluctant to leave a bed or bedroom, the activities director left and went on. I had no idea what the conversations were like, and I never had the chance to study the difference between invite and encourage.

When I asked my mom why she hadn't joined in coloring or jewelry making, she rolled her eyes and changed the subject. I was committed to uplifting her spirit, and I still thought she was fun, so I continued entertaining her—by default, I'd become her day camp counselor.

. . .

During her earlier time in independent living, I'd connected with my mom almost nightly. Sometimes, I attended the scheduled program: a recent movie, chamber music concert, or art lecture. On nights when I'd arrived after the events, she waited in her favorite upholstered chair in the lobby, greeting friends and holding court. We left the building and walked my dog around her long inner-city block, night after night, for three seasons— even in the rain.

My mother still dreamed of walking "with the girls" as she had during her Florida retirement, and sometimes another resident joined us, but our proud procession usually included my mom, her cane or walker, my dog, and me.

After she was confined to the assisted living wing, we continued our walks. When the hill around the senior living complex presented a challenge, we chose other, more level routes. If the weather was chilly, we walked through the complex's interior pathways: up a ramp that became increasingly difficult for her to negotiate, back to the once familiar dining and reception areas of the independent living buildings. My mom slowly lost interest in the world she'd once inhabited, but she longed to see and be seen by residents and staff who told her they missed her.

. . .

On Saturday mornings, during my mother's initial year in assisted living, a dedicated group of volunteers from the independent living apartments organized a weekly social hour in a remodeled area on the lowest floor of the assisted living wing. Staff members who accompanied most of the assisted living residents rarely stayed to observe or share the camaraderie. Volunteers served beverages, led friendly conversations, and sometimes displayed artifacts from their travels during sessions of show-and-tell. I included my little dog, and for an hour or more, we passed him from lap to lap, so each resident had a chance to cuddle him.

I added the Saturday-morning hour to our schedule. The atmosphere was convivial, and after months of uncertainty and disruption, I could relax for the precious moments when I saw my mom participating and talking to friends. Still, I was aware of how many unsafe events could occur in an unsupervised assemblage of fifteen or sixteen assisted living residents—from coughs and bathroom calls to confusion and falls.

At every juncture, with every day, I learned to be watchful for the neglect, errors, and unfortunate accidents that could further incapacitate my fragile mom—and further inconvenience me.

• • •

Once my mom moved from a CCRC near my home to facilities farther away, she lost nurturing connections with other Jewish residents and visitors. The nurse at her second assisted living facility celebrated Hanukkah and asked my mom to talk about recollections of growing up Jewish. The activities staff at her third facility led timely discussions about holidays like Passover and asked us to share matzoh as an afternoon snack.

Hospice notified the medical staff that my mother's spiritual needs should be supported within her care group. But she was the only Jewish resident in the unit.

My mom felt excluded from weekly prayer sessions and Bible readings that were unfamiliar to her. Religious hours that appeared on posted activities schedules disrupted her sense of belonging. When other residents gathered for weekly Bible study, hymn singing, or Communion, my mom sat alone.

As soon as my mother told me she was "different," I added additional hours to my care schedule. During prayers, I wheeled her to another part of the building—to her own room or outdoors if the weather was mild. In time, we met another Jewish woman, a former junior tennis champion, who lived in the independent living section and became a friend—by mutual attraction, not common religion.

• • •

When my able-bodied mother was still living independently, recent Hollywood releases played on a large screen in the CCRC entertainment area. Reading closed captions, she followed the plot—always telling me the acting was *superb*—and she had the ability to attend or leave at will. But, after her mobility was reduced by a stroke, and further diminished by a broken hip, my mom became stuck in one spot and relied on others to manage her access to viewing.

Accepted research and popular advice recommend stimulating the fading cognitive powers of people suffering from Alzheimer's and other dementias with gentle music, memory-generating images, and discussions about happy moments. Unfortunately, a combination of disinterest, low creativity, and long hours leads overworked and distracted caregivers to entertain residents with movies—elder-sitting by TV.

For decades, professional researchers have studied the number of hours toddlers and young children spend in front of screens, but we can only guess how harmful long days in front of TVs must be for older people, whether at home or in congregate settings. Eye strain and earaches from TV images and upturned volume are only the beginning. Sound barriers to socialization and uncensored streams of negative news frustrate efforts to calm anxieties and prepare residents for sleep. Still, mind-numbing screen watching remains an assisted living fact of life.

● ● ●

During her stay in her first assisted living home, the facility converted a suite on the lowest level into an area for movie viewing. One outspoken resident selected most of the movies from either Netflix or DVDs. A self-styled expert on world history, his choices were noticeably militaristic.

As soon as I realized my mother was being coaxed to move to the downstairs viewing space every evening, I started researching plot summaries on Wikipedia. I dissuaded her from attending movies that included domestic violence or gun battles. But when I tried discussing the appropriateness of certain story lines with the executive director, he invited me to his office and told me he couldn't be bothered—he didn't have time to read or care about movie synopses.

I sensed that the knowledgeable film buff was displaying symptoms of dementia, and I was sensitive to the adverse effect of his condition on my mom and her coresidents. Night after night, he claimed his favorite chair in the rear of the movie room, and, in a loud, intimidating voice, announced when he was ready for the film to start. He insisted that all slivers of ambient light be blocked out, and he told everyone to remain seated for the entire movie— even through the scrolling credits—until the final words, *The End.*

Many evenings, I stayed until I knew my mom was settled in her viewing spot, while my interest and concern bordered on anxiousness. She still retained the ability to stand and reach her walker, but if she'd chosen or needed to leave, she would probably have been incapable of navigating through the maze of chairs, walkers, and wheelchairs that were scattered between her and the only door.

Sometimes, caregivers wheeled attendees into the darkened room and turned to leave without noticing that the latecomers blocked the exit for everyone who'd assembled earlier. My concern turned to fear.

Once again, I approached the director, this time to inform him that because one resident insisted that all blinds be drawn to block the hallway light, caregivers who were passing by couldn't see into the interior of the room. Unobserved assisted living and memory care residents were effectively trapped in a crowded movie venue.

I was not surprised when the director responded that he didn't have sufficient staff to assign a responsible person to sit through full-length films with residents, but he agreed that one window shade along the wall should be raised several inches. Thereafter, caregivers had to remember to stoop in the adjoining hallway and peek into the darkened room as they walked by. As my fear for her safety increased, I began to build a case to transfer my mother to a smaller, more intimate assisted living facility.

Three nights before my mom moved out, *Zorba the Greek* was chosen as the evening's entertainment. When the activities director (the only staff member present) started the DVD, she began spinning to the opening music in a spirited Greek dance. She said, "This is how I spent my childhood." I didn't know if she meant she grew up in Greece or danced to lively folk music. After the opening scenes were played, she left.

I stayed in the room for the first half hour and began to recall that the plot contained dark twists. My mom indicated she wanted to stay, and I went home.

Two hours later, I received a call that my mother was frightened and frantic. When I spoke to her, she was still crying, "Why did they kill the old woman?" I felt more shame than anger and promised myself that I'd personally monitor future images my mom witnessed: no more violent mobs!

Later that night, one of the other assisted living residents wandered into my mom's room and frightened her again. I can't say whether the series of events was responsible, but by the following morning, my mother was limp and uncooperative—indicative of a ministroke. We spent six hours in the local emergency room. Two days later, I helped her move to her next assisted living facility.

• • •

While other caregivers were occupied with preparations for supper, the typically creative staff person at one of my mom's assisted living/memory care facilities arranged memory care residents around a TV and inserted one of two DVDs in the attached player: skits from Carol Burnett comedy shows or replays of the recently disgraced Bill Cosby's performances. I remember hearing the head nurse walk by and deliver a punch line from a Carol Burnett gag with perfect timing. The videos had played so many times that the caregiving staff had memorized the words!

Over and over, night after night, instead of planning a conversation or creative activity, staff people asked, "Do you want to watch a movie?" Without waiting for a response or even checking to learn what was in the DVD player, they wheeled immobile old people into a semicircle in front of a large flat-screen TV. *The King and I* and *Annie* were played so many times that my mother began to cry at the first notes. "Do not ever let them leave me in that room again," she said, and she meant it.

The underlying assumption seemed to be that the assembled residents didn't know or care. My mom, reacting to the ageist stereotyping, said, "They don't care. They know they're leaving us all alone and we can't do anything about it."

At my mom's fourth residence, less familiar films played twice a week. The residents knew when movie time approached. Leaving their rooms and personal TVs behind, they congregated by walker and wheelchair like fish in a tank, surfacing for a feeding. No one spoke, except during one movie that began with a love scene—when most of the group turned away and wheeled back to their rooms. Sometimes, one of the caregivers filled plastic cups with microwave popcorn. My mother never watched the films, and she couldn't swallow popcorn.

* * *

Wisconsin's Administrative Code requires every CBRF to conduct an entry assessment that becomes the template for each resident's individual service plan (ISP):

(1) Assessment.
> (a) Scope. The CBRF shall assess each resident's needs, abilities, and physical and mental condition before admitting the person to the CBRF, when there is a change in needs, abilities or condition, and at least annually. . . .
> (c) *Areas of assessment.* The assessment, at a minimum, shall include all of the following areas applicable to the resident: . . .

10. Social participation, including interpersonal relationships, communication skills, leisure time activities, family and community contacts and vocational needs.
> (d) *Assessment documentation.* The CBRF shall prepare a written report of the results of the assessment and shall retain the assessment in the resident's record.[33]

Six different CBRFs should have assessed my mom's level of social participation, but the collected data didn't translate into outcomes specific for her cognitive abilities, desires, and needs. Six

---

33. Wisconsin Administrative Code, Chapter DHS 83, "Community-Based Residential Facilities," Subchapter VII—"Resident Care and Services," DHS 83.35, "Assessment, individual service plan and evaluations."

times, whether responses were recorded in files, notebooks, or computer printouts, my mom was placed in the universal assisted living mix.

Sometimes the programming was appropriate for her physical, emotional, and mental condition, but more often, she was only a McResident. If she was bored or dozed off, or if she and her wheelchair were left on the other side of the room, she missed out.

• • •

Even after suffering a stroke and becoming immobile, my mother remained creative enough to join in poetry writing and spelling bees. When she added a phrase to a group poem or knew how to spell long words (she never lost the skill), she'd tell me about her achievement.

One creative activities coordinator organized challenging mind-stretching activities, but four of my mom's homes reduced her to the common denominator: bingo player. My mom never played bingo in her former life—she referred to it as "gambling." Still, when there was no other activity and she was awake, she learned to fill in a card or two, proudly challenging herself to locate the called numbers by herself—refusing prompting or assistance.

Some days my mom was tolerant and willing to join social or physical activities. Other days she was not. As time went on and she became weaker, she slept more often than she participated, and I spent longer hours watching her—typing my thoughts and observations long before I thought I'd be writing this book.

• • •

Sadly, immobility became a barrier. One morning, the director of the second assisted living facility told me my mom and several other residents had been transported to the second-floor craft room to make scrapbooks. When I looked around, I discovered she was still on the first floor—alone in her wheelchair. Apparently, the elevator had been full, and no one returned to retrieve her.

With limited space on one accessible van, my mother missed field trips that had previously delighted her, and, because the recently retrofitted van at another home still had no wheelchair safety straps, she wasn't allowed to ride along for sightseeing adventures or unplanned ice-cream parties. I responded by providing separate, but hopefully equal, diversions: my dog, a sunny location, and always the daily newspaper or books. When she entered her sixth home and had receded deep into her own world, I asked the staff for an activity apron (a colorful lap cloth sprinkled with buttons, zippers, Velcro, and various cloth textures), but by then, my dying mom lacked the minimal strength or interest to do anything but hold on.

• • •

Although her attention span steadily decreased, my mother wanted to read newspapers and magazines. Until she turned ninety-nine, she worked through the local paper in the morning and my print copy of *The New York Times* when she went to bed. She frequently surprised her caregivers by explaining or referring to articles she'd seen. As she approached one hundred, she lost interest, but she still looked at the front page, and she could tell me if she'd already seen the headlines.

When my mom became wheelchair-bound and couldn't access the community's copies, I began purchasing her own subscriptions. Day after day, I found her local paper neatly folded outside her room or on her dresser, where she couldn't see or access it. Some days, the paper was casually folded into the side pocket of her wheelchair. I had to recognize that a morning paper was not an important part of the young caregivers' daily existence, but for my mother, printed news and full-page ads connected her to her reality—and she was entitled to her own view of the world.

Before long, I gave up expecting that caregivers would hand a paper—with my mother's name written on it—to her. As soon as I arrived at her residence, I located her morning news (somewhere between the front desk in the lobby and her own bedside table) and tried to contribute current events and purpose to her day.

One of our friends brought semimonthly copies of the traditional Jewish magazine *Forward.* My mom looked at every page, column by column, and said, "The writing is marvelous."

By the time she moved to her sixth residence, my mother's attention span dropped to nil. After years of discussions about politics, inventions, and fashions, and after constant reminders about new products and local sales, I stopped leaving *The New York Times* on her blanket at night. I reluctantly canceled the recently renewed subscription to the daily local news.

• • •

Along with her fascination with reading and letters, my mother's preferred means of watching TV programs or movies was with the assistance of subtitles. While she was in independent living and her first assisted living home, subtitles were part of the culture. No one objected—unless they weren't turned on. As she moved to other assisted living facilities, managers who held no opinion or weren't trained in hearing and communication issues allowed residents and residents' families to switch off the closed captioning. I was especially disappointed when classic movies were on the schedule, accompanied by muted conversations, musical numbers, or foreign dialogue. The solution for caregivers seemed to be to turn up the volume—and the dissonance.

The usual staff response to requests for captioning was, "I don't know who turned it off," or "I don't know how to turn it on." Sometimes, I located remote-control devices and reinstalled subtitles myself, but that was not my job.

Eventually, as with many other concerns, I retreated. My mom had her own TV and cable connection. When we were cozy and sequestered in her room, she could watch TV with subtitles—often asking me the meaning of words she read, such as *cyberhack*. Once, she surprised me by saying, "I keep reading about Al-Qaeda. Why don't we ever see a picture of him?"

* * *

Only one residence offered calming background music. The executive director at my mother's third place, a trained classical violinist, selected light classical pieces or jazz melodies to air over the facility-wide sound system. Four months into my mom's tenure, he left, and the soft music ended. In four other facilities, small boom boxes appeared—sometimes brought by the caregivers themselves. One "life-enhancement coordinator" contributed a single Frank Sinatra CD. She pushed PLAY when she left for the day, and the tunes started to loop endlessly. Often, I appointed myself the sound police and lowered the volume or hit the STOP button, but, like closed captioning, endlessly repeating tunes should not have been my problem to solve.

My aging mother required less and less attention to respond with a quick smile. But, like many of her peers, if she wasn't constantly engaged, she drifted away and found solace in her own world. If a staff person distributed song sheets or projected words on a large screen, my mom could follow and sing along to familiar songs. Even as her voice became a dull monotone, she would speak—then, later, mouth—the words. Craving and appreciating attention, she asked for guidance from the facility's activities personnel: where to look in the songbooks and what page to read.

During a weekly piano sing-along with one beloved activities staff person, my mom began to share memories of her childhood and even recalled the name of the piece she practiced and would have played for her first piano recital, at age eleven—the week her mother (my grandmother) died. I somehow remembered that my mother had worn her new recital dress to the funeral, but I never focused on the piece she'd have played. I will remain forever grateful to our beautiful friend for eliciting the details of my mother's trauma.

● ● ●

When she lost her ability to stand and take charge of the floor, my mom, the lifelong performer, stopped reacting to dance music. Of course, there was a generational divide: For my mother, dance music meant the swing and big band era of the 1930s and 1940s, but for her caregivers and life-enhancement coordinators, dance music was louder, more rhythmic, and more contemporary. Behind her door, on long afternoons, I connected my iPhone to a Bluetooth receiver, and we survived in our own audio zone—a safe, familiar music island.

I sensed that unfamiliar music increased the confusion, agitation, and anxiety common to my mother's diagnosis of vascular dementia. The issue wasn't why she preferred a specific genre. The issue was that she not be subjected to sounds that were annoying and jarring to her—sounds that were amplified by her sensitive hearing aids. Without realizing it, as I wheeled her into her own room and played her preferred sounds, I was applying recognized music therapy.

The state had experimented with a Music and Memory program of individualized music delivered via headphones "to improve the care of residents with dementia and decrease the use of harmful medications." Trained caregivers created personalized music playlists, and the selections were delivered on digital devices. According to the Music and Memory website, "These musical favorites tap deep memories not lost to dementia and can bring participants back to life, enabling them to feel like themselves again, to converse, socialize and stay present."[34] Started in nursing homes, the program was reportedly adopted by assisted living communities, including my mother's third facility, but, to my knowledge, music therapy was never offered to my mom.

• • •

As we spent winter hours in her room, she in her ever-present wheelchair, comforted by bright pillows and a blanket, and I typing on my laptop computer, our time together became more intimate. Whether my mother dozed or remained awake, she appeared happier and more social in her cozy cocoon. As I relied less on staff to occupy or divert my frail mom, we all benefited.

But while I was discovering the therapeutic effects of classical, light jazz, and ballroom music, my mom's medical team (in consultation with hospice) was already prescribing antipsychotic medications. I countered by trying to control the staff's temptation to dose at will—or repeatedly increase the strength of her drugs.

I remained on alert for outbursts typical to OCD and sundowning that make any group or social activity impossible. At any moment, but more likely before or during dinner or at bedtime, my mother would become stuck on a single idea or subject with annoying tenacity: We had to take the dog out; she had to call the doctor; she had to make a grocery list for a holiday meal; she had to buy black shoes for her new black outfit; or she had to pay a bill. My mom expressed fears about losing or not having things she might need: her pocketbook, money, Kleenex, her eyeglasses, her comb—or, of course, the dog. She became afraid that her door or windows had been left open or her lights had been left on. At first,

---

34. https://www.dhs.wisconsin.gov/music-memory/index.htm.

she sounded cute, and her requests seemed manageable, but before long, she appeared restless, frustrated, and impossible to distract. She displayed erratic mood swings, became agitated, and demanded freedom from her restraints.

I watched, helplessly, as my unhappy mom tried to slip out of her wheelchair or pull off her transfer belt or sweater—as she began swinging her arms or feet, even as people were trying to help. Of course, I became the frequent target of sundown-induced angst. Within seconds, she changed her view of me—from her support-ive daughter to the person who'd brought her there to die. As she lost control, every aspect of her environment that was troublesome became more so: boredom, people she didn't recognize, claustro-phobia, and loneliness.

I attempted to present familiar games, books, or magazines, and, as the seasons passed in her various homes, we lengthened our late-afternoon wheelchair walks. Sometimes, the only activity that worked was backing off and waiting for the restoration of sanity—an old-fashioned time-out.

As she approached one hundred years of age, physicians and nurses continued experimenting with medications—some psycho-tropic and some narcotic—seemingly by trial and error. To pre-vent my ninety-pound mother from hurting herself, another resident, a caregiver, or *me*, I watched her swallow the frightening chemicals I'd previously resisted.

Instead of diversions, entertainment, and activities, I'd come to accept safety, comfort, and quiet sleep. In time, I stopped expecting our payments to cover creative distractions—the life-enhancing events promised by marketing brochures and websites—and I shed my overriding guilt about my failure to keep my mom active during her waking hours.

I made an uneasy, unforeseen peace with the assisted living industry that was far different from what we'd originally expected:

I continued paying monthly fees for monotonous security. In return, we received precious mother-daughter togetherness.

• • •

Over time, I came to appreciate gardens as meditative areas. When green spaces weren't planted or maintained, we sought our own. At her second assisted living place, I wheeled my mother through a nearby city trail with a preserved wetland area. I could spot herons and egrets as she watched tree colors change with the seasons.

While she lived in her third facility, we visited the gardens in a tiny public park across from the police station, and my mom never missed the private plantings along the way. If the patios surrounding the complex became crowded and noisy, we moved to a secluded spot at the end of the building. A retention pond provided a pretty view, and, occasionally, ducks appeared.

Over the course of my mom's last summer, at the ultimately unfriendly fourth site, we sat in a small front yard, where I read out loud while one other resident joined us. One August day, we found a space in front of a gas station and food mart across the highway. Because a friend had come to visit, we sat at a tiny picnic table, shared stale cookies, and watched traffic—creating our own respite in the filtered sunlight.

One week before my mother died, I noticed that the facility's staff were planting seeds in soil packed into paper cups—to transfer to an outdoor garden in warmer weather. I wheeled my calm companion to a round table in the activity area, and we began considering the project. A caregiver approached us and interrupted our springtime reverie. He wasn't there to explain flower seeds; he asked if I'd please use one of the sharp sticks (intended for seed identification) to clean under my mother's nails.

My mother's precious hands, the hands that had welcomed and nurtured me, hugged my children, prepared meals for our small family and for large community parties, worn diamonds and white gloves—and planted flowers from Boston to West Palm Beach—were now so likely to swing out and forcibly push people away that caregivers refused to hold and clean them. I nodded my head, held back tears of loss, and performed as I'd been asked: I removed stubborn dirt from my mother's nails.

A few days later, I held those thin hands for my mom's last manicure—polishing with her favorite red shade, Revlon's Cherries in the Snow.

* * *

Reportedly, Pope Francis "used his own vulnerability to demand dignity for the aged in a world increasingly populated by them . . . trying to reshape modern society to be more hospitable to the old." He said, "the marginalization of the elderly—both conceptual and practical—corrupts all seasons of life, not just that of old age."[35] I knew my marginalized mom was missing out on interests that still might keep her animated—and I missed our former existence.

When an activity took place and my mother participated or even observed, she added an extra smile to our lives. We knew nothing about assisted living until she was there, so we made things up, crisis by crisis. Many days, I'd say, "I don't know how else to do this."

The owner of my mom's fourth facility told me we were not happy, and we left. The owners of her fifth assisted living home appeared to disapprove when we lingered alone in quiet spaces, but I was simply admitting our limitations. Working against the forces of physiological deterioration and impairment, I acknowledged my

---

35. Jason Horowitz, "Pope Makes His Frailty a Lesson in Compassion," *New York Times*, July 29, 2002.

mom's advancing age and her waning ability to appreciate her surroundings.

Jessica Mitford wrote, "Whether the narrow passageway to the unknown, which everybody must cross, will continue to be as cluttered and as expensive to traverse as it is today depends in the last analysis entirely on those travelers who have not reached it yet."[36] We had come to the point where nothing more—neither dollars nor attention—could smooth the passage.

By the time my mother entered her sixth congregate home, we were both too tired to linger in the room designated for group events. A resident handbook with phone numbers and an inflated activities list couldn't lure or distract us any longer. We both craved peaceful moments—preferably in the sun.

• • •

My mom's birthday was approaching—April 21, the same day as Queen Elizabeth's. I'd always loved my mother's birthday—even more than mine: Spring arrived, the trees leafed out, flowers returned, and my mother basked in good wishes. Her favorite cakes were the ones she brought to other people, inscribed, "It's my birthday, but you get the cake." My mother appreciated the gifts I wrapped for her, and sometimes I rewrapped items she'd given me, or I'd already given her—sparkly possessions that made us laugh because we cherished them.

For years, my mom received flower arrangements from her grandkids and me, and then sent photos taken in her living room in Florida or in her various retirement homes—once from a hospital room. My mom wanted to be pictured in the center of blooming love, and she held up big cards for her photographers—so we'd know she was signaling *Thank you*.

---

36. Jessica Mitford, *The American Way of Death* (New York: Simon & Schuster, 1963), p. 287.

In April 2017, the hospice team ordered a marble sheet cake, and we celebrated a ninety-ninth birthday with coresidents and caregivers in my mother's third assisted living dining room. One year and three moves later, I began to doubt we'd see flowers arrive from grandchildren or hang the HAPPY BIRTHDAY banner, but I still unpacked our collection of candles and party napkins.

I hoped for the gift of more days, and we received one at a time. In the end, we received nine days too few for us to participate in the ultimate assisted living advertising video. We never sang "Happy 100th Birthday, Nana Lil."

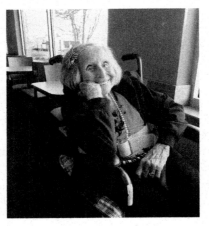

My mother, Lillian Deutsch, 2015.

Care Crisis

Demand for eldercare services has grown with the aging of the population, but the supply of trained, well-paid caregivers has not kept pace. The effects are being felt in home-care services and in congregate facilities. Turnover, inconsistent training, and the profitable temporary service industry are placing the burden on the wider community—and especially on families.

Adequate eldercare requires planning, but planning is often impossible. Until the week after my mother suffered a stroke, I had *no* care plan in place—no plan for her future. I didn't even know I was supposed to worry about it. I remained in denial because some things stayed the same: I took my dog to the hospital every morning, and he hopped onto her bed

I was involved in minute-by-minute details and couldn't think about the altered existence that waited outside the hospital walls.

The words *continuity of care* had a comforting ring, but I couldn't guess how, if, or when that would be achieved. Who would provide the care? I'd thought her age progression would evolve gradually, but I'd been wrong.

Hindering my mother's mobility, the black-and-blue hematoma covering her buttock since the bathroom fall, two weeks before, now reached to her waist. We assumed she'd struck something in her path when she fell in the night—while I was sleeping on her living room couch. Emergency room physicians at one hospital had sent her home with no diagnosis and no care instructions. Four days later, a second team of ER physicians, at a different hospital, had diagnosed a stroke and were, understandably, more concerned with stroke symptoms than butt bruises.

The day before she transferred from hospital bed to assisted living, a team of wound nurses appeared and, without explaining or suggesting future steps, crisscrossed my mother's bottom with multiple long strips of white adhesive tape. With that farewell gift, we left the now familiar routine of the stroke unit and began a confusing four-and-a-half-year odyssey that was intertwined with frequently unexplained, sometimes demeaning, and often demoralizing care.

● ● ●

Three sources of care interacted during my mother's final years:

1. Hospitals and ancillary specialty clinics

2. Assisted living facilities

3. Hospice

The hospital system included two affiliated entities—both had twenty-four-hour emergency rooms for which we could have been awarded frequent-user medals, had they existed. My mother's PCP was a member of the geriatrics staff of one of the hospitals. He performed regularly scheduled outpatient checkups until two months before she died. Every change in medications or procedures was reviewed and approved by the PCP.

Six assisted living facilities advertised themselves as locations for long-term care, but, by state code, they provided "not more than three hours of [nursing] care per week per resident."[37] Nonmedical assisted living attention, including help with dressing, toileting, meals, ambulation, and a varied schedule of activities—everything that occurred within a span of twenty-four hours—was provided by CNAs. Some CNAs-in-training, who provided less intense care, like food service, were high school students, often looking forward to careers in nursing. A noticeable number of CNAs were recent immigrants to the United States and new students of English. Surprisingly, many were related—mothers and daughters or aunts and nieces—and more than a few were men. Although well intentioned, they varied in interest and abilities, and all appeared underpaid; when one capable CNA abruptly left my mother's third residence, she sent us a message: "I'm sorry I quit. I miss you." I met her at her new job—serving at the drive-up window at Taco Bell.

A year and a half into our assisted living existence, hospice became integrated with my mother's care. From that point on, every change and decision bounced back and forth between the PCP or his nurse, the assisted living nurse, and the hospice nurse.

While each care component received or prepared to send phone or fax messages, my mom and I waited for clarifications and updates. If medication was involved, the local dispensing pharmacy that packaged doses for assisted living facilities also entered the discussion.

• • •

When I needed advice about a change in my mother's condition, I called her geriatric clinic and took my place in line: I listened to

---

37. "Choosing an Assisted Living Facility," State of Wisconsin, Department of Health Services, Division of Quality Assurance, Bureau of Assisted Living, p-60579 (Rev. 09/2012), p. 2.

the repetitive and too familiar *hold* melody, until I spoke to a person who screened all calls. If my question or request merited consideration, a nurse called me back. Because all decisions were made by the PCP, who maintained a full outpatient schedule, I couldn't receive a resolution or confirmation of new orders until after his clinic hours—usually after 4:00 P.M. Sometimes, when I was involved with my mother, I missed or didn't hear my cell phone. Then I hurried to call back—to reach the same nurse who'd called me—before 5:00 P.M., when the clinic switchboard shut down.

Orders from the PCP were faxed to the assisted living facility, and if the fax messages weren't received, noticed, or read soon enough, even longer delays occurred. Too often, the communications loop forced everyone involved to wait to update my mother's care (even changes in medications) until the following day.

Because my mother periodically suffered bouts of loose stools, even the simple need to increase her (already prescribed) loperamide dose meant calls to both the facility nurse and hospice—and eventually to her PCP. On my birthday in 2016, I was awakened by an early-morning call from a concerned caregiver: My mom's supply of loperamide had run out. I left my house before dawn and traveled to an all-night Walgreens to purchase over-the-counter pills. I continued to keep a contraband supply that I could administer myself, as needed—with the full knowledge of the CNAs, whose hands were tied.

For us, the dangerous flaw in the hospital/assisted living/hospice trifecta was the medicine order and distribution web. On the night my mom died, I realized I should have been more wary of the intricate communications trap that could collapse around us—leaving her without morphine, the common end-of-life prescription that would have assisted us through a merciful passage.

• • •

The afternoon my mother moved to assisted living, I gave all her medicines to the assisted living nurse. In the weeks when I was still moving furniture, recycling clothing, and clearing out her independent apartment, I was relieved to have help with meds. On the day the nurse confiscated over-the-counter eyedrops, I knew I'd yielded control forever.

In my mother's room at her first assisted living home, pills were stored in an upper cabinet, above a small sink. I remember a locked section, but I don't think any of her meds were kept in that secure area. Caregivers came by, presumably on schedule, and handed her pills and water.

In the residences that followed, I became aware that the medicine-distribution system was carried out by med passers dispensing pills from containers that were organized on wheeled carts. (At one facility, the assortment of pills and medications were housed in stationary cabinets outside the residents' rooms.)

Some CNAs were med passers, but not all med passers were CNAs. The Wisconsin rule says, "Unlicensed personnel are required to meet specific requirements to be able to administer medications to . . . nursing home residents and hospice patients." By state regulation, med passers are required to:

1. Be at least 18 years of age.
2. Have a high school diploma or high school equivalency diploma.
3. Be current on Wisconsin Nurse Aide Registry.
4. Be current on the federal nurse aide registry
5. Have at least 2,000 hours experience in direct patient care within the last three years.
6. Have worked a minimum of 40 hours within the last 90 days with residents receiving medications.
7. Be recommended in writing by the director of nursing and the administrator of the agency where you'll be working.

> 8. Be recommended in writing by two licensed charge nurses
> under whose licenses you'll be giving medications.[38]

I presumed the med passers received additional compensation. I knew they were performing serious tasks and respected that they shouldn't be distracted when they were dispensing meds. Still, I witnessed potentially dangerous inconsistencies.

As my mother grew older and her sundowning became more noticeable and difficult to manage, I started chasing down the afternoon med passers who worked in her third residence—trying to assure that she received her antianxiety pills. My mom had started suffering from coughing spells, and the hospice nurses had asked the facility to dispense her pills at 4:00 P.M., thereby allowing her time to "digest" them before her 4:30 dinner.

Night after night, I followed med passers around the meandering memory care unit. Sometimes they were busy with other residents, and I successfully reminded them to include my mother in their schedules. Often, I couldn't find them at all. The long-term care complex was a rambling structure, and scarce med passers could be sent to the adjoining RCAC section—just when I hoped they'd be available to help with my mom.

One night, a traveling med passer appeared—not from a staffing agency, but from a branch facility ninety miles away. She noticed me with my mother and asked *me* to identify the residents (I really didn't know them all), so she could distribute their pills.

During a confusing morning at her fifth assisted living facility, I noticed that my mother's pills were still in a paper cup on her dresser—not administered the night before. The most important responsibilities were left to the least well trained, and I saw how serious errors might occur.

---

38. Wisconsin Department of Health Services, "Medication aide programs and requirements," www.dhs.wisconsin.gov/regulations/nh/medaides -requirements.htm.

. . .

While my mom lived independently, and before she suffered a stroke and a broken hip, I regularly posted to my blog, *Mothers-GrownUpChild*. In a lighthearted mood, I often recorded adventures with hearing aids—her weapons of mass destruction (WMDs). The expensive high-tech items were frequently misplaced—and sometimes lost. I searched for them on the floor of a restaurant in a busy tourist area, in the cushions of the patio seating at her independent living apartments, and on the church steps of a neighboring Episcopal church—after an apparently homeless person told me he'd seen one there. (For the record: One aid was found at the church and another in the outdoor chair cushions, but a third was lost forever on the restaurant floor.)

My mother kept her own supply of batteries and recognized the telltale beep that reminded her she had to change them. Once she moved to assisted living, someone else had to check whether she was wearing the aids, whether the batteries were engaged, and whether the batteries were working.

If a CNA helped my mom to bed and forgot, didn't know, or neglected to remove the hearing aids, they'd fall into her bedding or beside her bed while she slept. If someone new or inexperienced helped her in the morning, that person had no idea my mother wasn't communicating because of lost or missing aids or batteries.

The solution was a carefully worded note beside my mom's bed and a description of the tiny battery cover that had to be opened when the aids weren't in her ears. New CNAs or temporary staffing agency CNAs routinely missed the note. They were helping an unfamiliar resident prepare for the day and didn't know or ask why she was silent.

Too often, I arrived partway through the day and noticed that my mother was particularly noncommunicative. I gradually realized we had hearing aid or battery problems. Everyone was blameless, but my frustration mounted. In those unexpected moments, I became aware I couldn't provide the detailed care I thought my mother deserved. Even now, I'm saddened by the silent, lost hours of alertness and my inability to improve her rapidly deteriorating assisted living existence.

* * *

My mom wanted to be loved. She hugged her caregivers—both nurses and CNAs. She asked about their families, and, when they were off duty, they brought their kids to meet her. More than anything, my mother wanted to hear about their partners, and she teased when she suspected that anyone might be planning to be married. (She was usually the first to know, and she was certain she would attend every wedding.)

One CNA in my mother's first facility returned every Sunday—on her day off—to accompany my mom on a walk through the complex, taking her to a window on the top floor of the independent living section so that they could look at the view over the city and lakes. Every Sunday: my mother with her walker and her devoted young friend.

When she started to forget caregivers' names, my mother asked me to write them down for her, in big letters. Each time she moved, I ordered new calling cards—pretty flowers with her name, room number, and facility. My mom, the former corporate executive, wanted to be known and recognized. She kept the cards in a china dish on her dresser and never forgot to hand them out: "Here, please take my card!"

With her Boston accent and propensity for puns, she made her CNAs laugh. After the morning assistants began braiding her hair and attaching bows, my mom told them they were spelled *B-E-A-U-S*. Then she'd add, "Get it?" My mother had her favorites, and she was the favorite of many. One February morning, she woke to a room door decorated with her name, dozens of red hearts, and congratulations for being selected as the assisted living staff's Valentine's Sweetheart.

Ever socially aware, my mom made plans to "go out for dinner" with her helpers, and she always included me—alas, the dinners never happened. When my daughter jogged or biked to visit her grandmother, they spent hours making lists of items needed for the next party: paper plates, napkins, crackers, cheese, soft drinks . . .

Sadly, but importantly, my mother recognized those who ignored her or others. She'd look at someone and tell me, "She's not sincere." Before long, we became affected by the chronic short-term nature of assisted living caregivers' commitments. One after another, CNAs came to tell us they were transferring to other facilities (usually for higher pay), returning to school, or leaving the care industry all together.

When long-term care became short-term care, we were both affected. I explained meal preferences, transfer abilities, and clothing needs to new personnel several times a week. A longtime friend and retired physician met me for lunch and diagnosed my exhaustion as "caregiver fatigue." Still, I became ever more cautious about trusting my mother's care to strangers.

On an afternoon when we returned to my mom's third home from a dental visit, I called ahead to the nurses' station to say we were parking at the closest door. I asked for assistance with a transfer from car to wheelchair. My mom was uncomfortable and wanted to use the bathroom, but no one appeared. Leaving her in the car (a bad idea, since she could open the door), I hurried into the building. Three CNAs, wearing pink uniforms from a local staffing agency, were sitting in a row near the TV-watching area. They ignored my request for help, and one said to the others, "She doesn't like agency." They had it right, because I was opposed to the inconsistency of temporary employment, but they had me cornered and were not planning to lend a hand.

I found the head nurse, who helped me remove my mother from my vehicle. Realizing I was asking for something that was unusual—and since there was no chain of command—I let the matter drop.

. . .

Beyond caregiving attitude, we had a regional communication problem. An aging woman who'd grown up in New England had been transported to the Midwest. "Have you ever been to Boston?" she asked everyone she met. Intending to be engaging, she often struggled to be understood. On a day when the hospice nurse reported that my mom was happy and thankful for the visit, she also reported that my mom's "speech continues to worsen, at times unable to understand her at all."

Of course, worker-patient exchanges were further complicated by caregivers who were new to the state or to the United States and spoke with unfamiliar accents. Sadly, underprepared personnel was not a recent problem. In the year 2000, a Minnesota hospital phoned an assisted living facility about a recently admitted patient. When no one responded, the hospital called the local police. "An officer was sent to the facility, where an aide who spoke almost no English answered the door. . . . The officer found just two other staff members, neither of whom spoke English well."[39]

I spent as much time as I could comforting, accompanying, and interpreting. What began as a family game (only I could interpret her words) became an emotional drain. I knew I needed a break, and I heard people who loved us tell me to leave: "Why can't you just go home early, Judy?" But I couldn't think of any

---

39. Andrew Goldstein/Eagan, "Better than a Nursing Home?" *Time*, August 13, 2001.

other way to hold things together than to be present—constantly present.

On her part, my formerly highly socialized mom was reluctant to welcome hospice volunteers. However, over a three-month period at her third facility, one persistent hospice visitor gradually earned my mother's acceptance. At first, the volunteer tried chatting and reading, but my mother only wanted to talk about waiting for me. Then, when the volunteer heard my mom say she was unhappy in her surroundings, she took her for a wheelchair stroll, and was surprised to see how many people knew Lillian as friendly. When my mother wanted to sleep, the volunteer simply stayed with her. When my mother waved her away, the volunteer wrote that she would keep trying. Unsurprisingly, one of their most meaningful exchanges was when my mother was seated at the dining room table with another resident—a man. (We could almost always count on my mother to become talkative and flirt.) In a gift to me, the volunteer noted: "Lillian was in good spirits today. I sat with her while she had a snack. She is beginning to recognize me and is more open to visiting. . . . Lillian is now happy to see me. She gave me a kiss on the hand!!!"

But direct caregivers rarely had time to be persistent or patient. Often, they abruptly encircled my mom's slight frame and lifted or nudged her into her wheelchair or dining room seat. Recurring hospice notes describe falls and slowly healing leg bruises, but they also include my requests to transfer my mother's aging body *gently* with a gait belt. As with other accessories, both decorative and essential, I'd ordered gait belts in several colors. One nurse wrote that I was "very adamant" that a gait belt be worn for all transfers.

In July 2015, after my mom suffered a ministroke in her second residence, the facility nurse and hospice nurses agreed I could start looking for a pivot disc, a device that allowed her to stand firmly while her assistant (I was the assistant) guided her—with a gait belt—to turn ninety degrees from her position in front of one chair (or toilet) to a position in front of another chair (or wheelchair).

Although I later became aware that Medicare would reimburse hospice for a pivot disc that hospice would deliver to us, I ordered one from Amazon. When the new tool arrived, I wrote my mom's name on the back in oversized yellow letters. We held two practice sessions in the common hallway, outside my mother's door: the hospice nurse, the facility nurse, my mom, and I. Eventually, additional caregivers performed the transfers, but I did not take on the responsibility of trainer.

I created a side pocket in the wheelchair, so the disc was always available, and we became the synchronized dance team my mother dreamed about: *Stand. Hold on to me. I'll do the turning. Sit.* Forever the entertainer, she would kiss my cheek mid-transfer or smile and wave to her imaginary crowd.

We employed the pivot disc for almost three years—until the day my failing mom was admitted for her last hospital stay. When the hospital staff cited liability concerns and refused to allow us to perform transfers as my mother had been taught, she lost the ability to balance or participate. My mother became a prisoner of a demeaning and relatively unsafe mechanical Hoyer lift for the last seven weeks of her life.

• • •

As she entered each new facility, my mom was shown a way to announce that she needed assistance. Aware of her own needs, but increasingly incapable of helping herself, she received call buttons, or fobs, that she wore around her neck like signature pieces of jewelry. (At her fourth home, the only way to alert caregivers was to pull a ribbon attached to an outdated call system attached to the bedroom wall.)

My mother learned quickly that response time could be uncomfortably long, especially if she had to use the toilet—particularly if she was not in her room. With the agreement and approval of the director of her fourth residence, I purchased a remote doorbell from Home Depot and glued it to a wheelchair cushion.

When my mother pushed the doorbell button, a loud ringing occurred in the corner where caregivers congregated—usually to prepare medications. After a short while, someone unplugged the ringer because the sound was disruptive—as it was intended to be—and because my mother was the only resident with a bell. My creative problem solving was not recognized or appreciated. I donated the device to my mother's next facility (her fifth), where an outside button might still be alerting caregivers that someone is awaiting entrance at the locked front door.

• • •

At her initial assisted living residence, while she was still mobile, my mom had been frightened by an alarm that was triggered if any resident tried to open a hallway door after hours. One night, she was so scared that she left her bed, reached under a tall dresser, and disconnected the plug on her own TV. The plug wasn't the source of the noise, and her action should have been a red flag for us all. The director of the facility moved the dresser closer to the wall, so my mom could no longer reach the electric outlet, but no one talked about my mother's fears—or her abrupt, unsafe actions.

After my mom broke her hip and would never walk again, she was found on the floor countless times. She wanted to leave her bed and thought she was able to do so, but she could no longer be trusted to be left alone. When my mother started rolling out of her bed at naptime, the nurse in her second residence and I finally agreed: no daytime snoozing in her private bedroom. Because her elaborate wheelchair could be tilted back far enough for my mom to recline, even to nap, she remained in her wheelchair for all her waking hours—stuck in the common areas, where someone could observe her.

My mother grew impatient. She let the staff know she was not happy with the responses to her requests for help. Busy caregivers told her they had many people to care for, and they were doing the best they could. One nurse wrote, "Pt [patient] stated she didn't want them promising that they would be right back and they never show up."

She'd become a danger to herself. Many nights, she was found on the floor, usually without injury. One direct caregiver acknowledged, "She did call several times through the night, but when she called the last time, staff went to her room, and she was already on the floor."

Even if I'd stayed with her 24/7, I would not have been able to protect her. She'd stare at me and say, "I saw two big doctors [for her, they were always *big* doctors] and they both said I could walk."

● ● ●

One week before she turned ninety-eight, she was found on the floor between the bathroom and her bed at 10:45 P.M. A caregiver noted, "She had likely been trying to walk to the bathroom on her own." A more accurate guess would have been that my mother had somehow rolled out of bed onto the floor, and she had tried to crawl toward the toilet. She could *neither stand nor walk.*

Two and half weeks later, hospice was summoned during the night—an unscheduled visit due to another unwitnessed fall. When the hospice nurse tried to arouse my mother with a light touch to her arm, she asked, "What are you doing here?" She claimed the fall had occurred a long time before. (Indeed, many falls had occurred over a long while.) When the hospice nurse attempted to examine her and asked if the palpation of her spine caused pain, my mother's response was, "Of course it does, you woke me up!"

My guess is that my mother needed to use the toilet and could not wait until a caregiver appeared. When the executive director told me he ran a busy facility, and the anticipated response time to a resident's call button alert was twenty minutes, I thanked him for his honesty.

• • •

Three years before she died, I'd helped an elderly woman who was recuperating from hip surgery return to an assisted living facility where she received infrequent PT. The sad results were that my mom spent her remaining days in what became a series of stiff metal frames on wheels. Just as I'd named my mother's hearing aids the "WMDs," her wheelchairs could have been called her "battering rams." I never knew anything about walkers or wheel-chairs, but I became proficient in assembling, disassembling, repairing, maneuvering, and adjusting things that rolled. We experimented with wheelchairs that offered various safety and comfort features, and soon my mom had new items to collect— toddler-size pillows in bright patterns that we arranged to cushion her tired arms and weakened back.

Although some wheelchairs were provided by Medicare (via hospice), at the time of my mom's death, we owned three models, which I donated (along with a full array of mobility equipment) to local nonprofit agencies.

The battering ram scenario was cued whenever my mother required transferring into and out of her wheelchair. The maneu-ver required clearing an area for a nonwalking person to pivot or be pivoted, which meant that both wheelchair footrests had to be detached *every single time*. (Simply loosening them was ineffective and dangerous: If they were merely swung to the sides of the chair, they were free to swing back and injure either the attending caregiver or my mom.)

Removing the heavy, unwieldy metal components was tricky. Even after three years of multiple transfers per day, I was sometimes incapable of holding each footrest precisely in place long enough to remove or reattach it with either speed or grace. While I fumbled, kneeling awkwardly beside the chair, my mother still had to go to the toilet, be seated at the dining room table, or be moved into a recliner for a nap.

We were all challenged by the poorly designed devices that had the potential to inflict serious harm. When caregivers either overlooked or didn't know how to remove and replace wheelchair footrests, my mom's paper-thin skin became bruised.

I received messages that my mother had sustained "unwitnessed" wounds on her lower legs. I knew that most of the lacerations were caused by unstable knifelike objects that could cut her while she was being transferred. My mom, whose articulation had diminished, knew she might be hurt, but she couldn't protect herself by explaining the necessary steps:

1. Deliver chair (with passenger) to desired space.

2. Lock chair.

3. Lift one metal footrest to exactly the right angle, where it can be eased away.

4. Remove footrest.

5. Repeat, for second footrest.

6. Move both unwieldy metal footrests *away* from the path of the transfer.

7. Accomplish the transfer task (to toilet, couch, chair, or car).

8. When ready, repeat steps 1–7, in reverse.

Caught between her immediate needs and painful transfers, my mom started resisting help and reacting against her caregivers—especially new and unfamiliar ones. Although confined to her wheelchair, she still possessed upper-body strength, and she could push people away (including me). Even though her words were frequently garbled and difficult for new caregivers to understand, she retained the ability to use her mouth. When she was agitated over waiting for eventual care, my mother started trying to bite those closest to her. Surprised staff members sometimes thought she was having a seizure, but with with patience and the attention she craved, she could still be talked down.

Well-intentioned nurses instinctively applied antibiotic ointments and bandages to the assorted wounds on my mom's legs. After months of observing, we learned the only way her skin tears would scab over was by exposure to the air—preferably, to the sun. Whenever a new nurse or hospice caregiver appeared and reapplied standard dressings, we had to begin the healing process all over again.

I intervened, advocated, and backed off. I couldn't train every caregiver in wheelchair mechanics, because that wasn't my responsibility; I couldn't train every nurse about wound care for a specific body—that wasn't my responsibility, either. I certainly couldn't be present to perform every task, but, whenever I could, I dressed my mother's wounds myself—removing gooey coverings, opening the affected areas to the air, and applying clean, dry coverings when protection was warranted.

*   *   *

My mom had moved to her first assisted living facility when she required help showering, eating, and taking medications. As time went on, she needed help with dressing, mobility, and toileting. Eventually, she required near-constant observation, assistance with all transfers, and sleep monitoring.

Depending on the time of day, my mom was either wheelchair-bound or bedridden, and she willed herself to be out of her restraints. Bathroom waits, transfer scenarios, and frequent skin wounds wore her down. The hospice notes started including action words: "fighting, spitting, pinching, biting, pulling hair," as well as the assessment: *agitated*. We were living with someone who wanted to be understood, and we were living with dementia.

In highly regarded assisted living facilities dedicated to the care of elderly people with declining capabilities, my mother sensed danger. Only a few staff members were willing or patient enough to interpret her reactions as calls for help.

At her third facility, early-morning caregivers told me they'd found my mom on the floor with soggy newspapers strewn about. I suspected my mother had to use the toilet during the night. When she'd waited long enough for a caregiver, she tossed her copy of *The New York Times* onto the floor, somehow lowered herself from the bed, and used the newspaper to try to scoot across the carpet toward the bathroom.

But my ingenious and frustrated mom never arrived at the bathroom; she wet herself and the newspapers on the floor. When I pieced together what had happened, I asked her, and she panto-mimed her actions by pumping her arms, as she would have had to do while slithering on her butt toward the toilet. Even if she'd made it to the toilet, she never could have lifted her body to the seat.

My mother had urinated on her beloved *Times*—on the floor of a room that was designed to provide her with dignity, independence, and care. The plaque at the entrance to the unit honored the matriarch of the business's founding family: "We calibrated what we did as a family to create a culture that protected her dignity while encouraging her independence." But somewhere, the noble care commitment had been lost.

• • •

At her fifth facility, the concerned owners placed an alarm under her sheets, but my curiously agile mother still managed to slip out. When she had only weeks to live, my daughter and I watched my mom fall asleep in a low bed in her final room. In her dream state, she gracefully danced through the motions of leaving her bed, never opening her eyes.

A novelist working on a memoir about her mother wrote, "There is wisdom and humor and radiance here if we look for it."[40] Sadly, few looked for it beyond our family, our close friends, and me. Dementia was not who she was, but, without staff support, I struggled to see what care remained beneficial. I might have set out on an unachievable quest, but I continued to seek *understanding*.

My gregarious and gracious mom, who'd opened our home to her widowed father and returning World War II veteran brother, and who hugged friendly people on any occasion, now had a virtual PROCEED WITH CAUTION sign around her. She became a pariah, and—by blood—I was a member of her caste.

• • •

On my mother's birthday, two years after she passed, a journalist and observer of the retirement years wrote, "The pandemic has given new urgency." Citing the "existential problem for facilities for older adults: People don't want to live there, don't want to work there, and don't want to place their parents there." He noted that "more than 400,000 workers at long-term care facilities [had] left the profession."[41]

---

40. Suzanne Finnamore, "Dementia Is Where My Mother Lives. It Is Not Who She Is," *New York Times*, May 11, 2022.
41. John Leland, "Can Robots Save Nursing Homes?" *New York Times*, April 21, 2022.

Emily K. Abel, professor emerita at the Fielding School of Public Health, UCLA, wrote, "Because vulnerability and dependence are inescapable features of all human life, caregiving is an essential activity that deserves greater recognition and support."[42] Left unaddressed, our care crises will only worsen, and underdiscussed flaws in the assisted living industry will continue to render care both haphazard and unsafe, while staff deployment approaches exploitation.

We still have the power to formulate the discussion and redefine eldercare. We can begin to downplay profits and establish the framework for a truly American system that honors direct care workers, families, and the elderly.

---

42. Emily K. Abel, *Elder Care in Crisis: How the Social Net Fails Families* (New York, New York University Press, 2022), p. 175.

Hospice

Specialized care for the dying was introduced to the United States in 1963, when Yale University's then dean Florence Wald invited Dame Cicely Saunders of the UK to participate in a visiting lecture at Yale. Four years later, in 1967, Saunders created St. Christopher's Hospice in the UK. Then, in 1974, Florence Wald founded Connecticut Hospice in Branford, Connecticut—America's first hospice.

Within five years and after several national conferences, the U.S. Department of Health, Education and Welfare acknowledged that hospices provided alternative care programs for Americans losing their lives to terminal illnesses. A report to Congress, prepared in 1978, at the request of Senators Abraham Ribicoff of Connecticut, Edward M. Kennedy of Massachusetts, and Robert J. Dole of Kansas, found fifty-nine organizations that considered themselves to be hospices, and seventy-three others being planned.[43]

---

43. Comptroller General of the United States, Report to the Congress of the United States, *Hospice Care—A Growing Concept in the United States*, U.S. General Accounting Office, Washington, D.C., March 6, 1979, front cover.

There is no standard definition of a hospice or of what services an organization must provide to be considered a hospice. However, in the United States, the hospice concept generally is considered to be a program that provides palliative care—medical relief of pain—and supportive services to terminally ill persons and assistance to their families in adjusting to the patient's illness and death.[44]

Federal hospice regulations were drafted: In 1982, Medicare added hospice care to its benefits, and in 1985, Medicare hospice coverage became permanent.[45] By 2015, when my mom was enrolled for services, there were 1.4 million patients in over four thousand U.S. care agencies[46]; in 2018, when my mother was reenrolled for the last month of her life, 1.55 million Medicare beneficiaries were receiving hospice services and supplies.

At that time, the average end-of-life length of stay was 89.6 days, and 53.8 percent of Medicare beneficiaries received care for thirty days or less. "A principal diagnosis of cancer (29.6 percent) was the leading diagnosis among Medicare hospice patients, followed by principal diagnosis of circulatory/heart disease (17.4 percent) and dementia (15.6 percent)."[47] In March 2022, *The Washington Post* described hospice as "an interdisciplinary

------

44. Comptroller General of the United States, Report to the Congress of the United States, *Hospice Care—A Growing Concept in the United States,* U.S. General Accounting Office, Washington, D.C., March 6, 1979, p. i.

45. "Most observers agree the primary motivation was to transfer care work to families in order to contain health care costs. Alarmed by the amount of government money spent on caring for elderly people in the final months of life, legislators were eager to find a way to reduce that expense." Emily K. Abel, *Elder Care in Crisis: How the Social Net Fails Families* (New York: New York University Press, 2022), p. 95.

46. *Long-Term Care Providers and Services Users in the United States, 2015–2016,* Appendix III.

47. National Hospice and Palliative Care Organization, *NHPCO Facts and Figures,* August 17, 2020.

approach that prioritizes comfort and quality of life in a person's final months."[48]

. . .

Despite common belief, hospices are not run by volunteers. Volunteers might become part-time visitors or assistants for a variety of tasks, but hospice administrations are led by professionals who are evaluated on financial performance and organizational viability. Hospice care is free to recipients and families and available at all income levels, but hospices are *businesses,* and they must raise sufficient funds through donations, gifts, bequests, and reimbursements to compensate employees, repay loans, cover operating costs, and plan for exigencies.

Whether structured as for-profit or nonprofit entities, hospices rely on Medicare reimbursements for patient services, medications, and supplies. In 2020, two years after my mother's death, Medicare paid for 85.4 percent of all hospice costs; Medicaid, 5 percent; private insurance, 6.9 percent; and charity and self-pay, 2.9 percent.[49]

In time, I learned that Medicare payments to a hospice agency are disallowed if a patient's prognosis indicates that life expectancy will exceed six months. I also learned that age per se is not considered a terminal illness, and neither is vascular dementia, because it does not progress in a predictable manner.

. . .

In my midwestern city, a nonprofit hospice organization had been in existence for four decades. They were known and respected for

48. Emily Harris, "For End-Stage Dementia, Medicare Can Make Hospice Harder to Access," *Washington Post,* March 26, 2022.
49. www.hospicenews.com/2020, December 16, 2020.

providing hospice services to people who were aging, seriously ill, or dying, as well as grief support for families and loved ones. They advertised that were "caring every step of the way."

Three months after my mother suffered a broken hip and was clearly not going to walk again, the resident nurse at her second assisted living facility arranged a time for us to meet with the hospice marketing team. We both listened, but neither of us heard any reason to sign up.

When I realized that my mom's medications would be evaluated and likely be reduced, and that she'd no longer be eligible for Medicare-funded physical therapy (even though still rehabilitating from hip surgery), I said, "No." I was told that the facility's nurse reacted by saying I didn't always make the best decisions for my mother, and I started to wonder whether signing up a hospice patient benefited the assisted living facility staff, because they'd have fewer tasks and responsibilities—while charging the same fees.

After my mom completed her allotted PT sessions, we received a second visit from the hospice marketing team. A discussion arose about biweekly showers from hospice aides who could relieve the assisted living facility staff (whom we'd continue to pay for in-house showers, per contract). My mother's days were becoming less stimulating, and she could look forward to being pampered by regularly scheduled showers. We said, "Yes."

On April 7, 2015, my mother was admitted to the routine home level of care for comprehensive interdisciplinary hospice services. She was cooperative and content. We felt she'd be well cared for, and we both felt calm.

• • •

Welcome, nonintrusive changes occurred: A reduced assortment of medications—in dose-controlled bubble packs—arrived daily from the long-term care branch of a local pharmacy; my mom received incontinence supplies (adult diapers), an endless variety of body wipes, lotions, certain over-the-counter medications— including cough syrup—and a wheelchair.

My mother was cautious about visits from hospice volunteers, asking why *she* had to entertain *them*, but she accepted biweekly showers from hospice staff and regular visits from a team of hospice nurses and a social worker. There seemed to be coordination between the assisted living facility nurse and the hospice organization's visiting nurses, and I received an email report after every scheduled visit.

Because hospice care focuses on maintaining rather than regaining strength, and Medicare no longer covered my mother's physical therapy sessions, we contracted privately with a personal trainer, who visited weekly and led her through simple wheelchair movements. She remained compliant and engaged; when the trainer asked, "You're not holding your breath are you?" she responded, "I can't afford to."

Although I didn't contact them for a while, the hospice call center was available 24/7. The third branch of the care tree (PCP/residence/hospice) was in place.

The hospice marketing team left a selection of proprietary and general reading material, including discussions on personsal dignity and confidentiality, do not resuscitate (DNR) information, and an advance planning guide. One page was clear about eligibility requiring a life expectancy of six months or less, but I didn't process the statement, because my mother did not have a life-limiting condition.

After a few weeks, the director of the assisted living facility told me again that people who were in hospice were expected to die within six moths. I stared at her with tears in my eyes. I had accepted the concept of comfort over cure, but I hadn't understood that we were signing up for impending death, and, indeed, my mother lived almost three years longer.

Day after day, I spent time at my mom's side, helping her eat, dress, and access the toilet. Night after night I washed and dried her laundry in my own basement and went to bed, relieved that I had nighttime coverage—not only the overnight staff at the facility but also the twenty-four-hour hospice line.

• • •

I was sound asleep at 2:58 A.M. on Monday, May 18, 2015, when my cell phone rang. A hospice nurse woke me and said, "I'm calling to tell you that your mother has died." She used no euphemisms. She didn't say *passed* or *passed away*. She said *died*. I was shaken out of a sound sleep—the sleep everyone said I needed. After the caller said, "I'm sorry to have to be the one to tell you," I managed to ask, "Did she struggle?"

I tossed off the covers and began taking one step at a time. I wondered if it was wise to call my kids in the middle of the night and tried to remember which one lived in which time zone.

At 2:59 A.M., the phone rang again. Expecting to hear either the director or the nurse from my mother's second assisted living facility, I immediately said, "I know." Unimaginably, the same voice I'd just heard said, "I'm so sorry . . . I called the *wrong number*. I'm at a different facility and I had the wrong file."

I never fell back to sleep. I kept thinking I should leave my house and drive through the dark night to hold my mom.

The next morning, I awakened to an email message expressing deep apology. The hospice employee repeated what she'd said on the phone: She'd accessed the wrong chart when attempting to notify a different family. She apologized for waking me and adding stress to my life. In closing, she added that I was a "devoted daughter" and that the relationship between my mother and me warmed her heart.

Five and a half weeks later, I received a message on an official letterhead. A senior staff member thanked me for providing feedback for the phone incident. She included a second apology and a pledge to identify ways to prevent similar situations in the future.

A hospice nurse had called in the middle of the night and said my mother had *died*. The communications used the words *shocking news, a situation,* and *this experience*. No one ever looked at me to say it was a careless, incompetent, unprofessional error. No one erased the words that reverberated in my head: "I'm sorry to have to be the one to tell you."

I don't know if you grieve someone only once, but I know that, from that moment, I was constantly on alert. I trusted no one. I continued to interact with hospice personnel and nurses and with professional staff in four other assisted living facilities and two hospitals. Stumbling from peaceful moments to periods of disappointment and conflict, I struggled to keep my emotional balance for the next three years.[50]

*   *   *

I began to realize we needed help beyond the basic assisted living model. Caring or advocating for my mother meant acknowledging her specific needs:

1. Psychological: Her fear, loneliness, and obsessive-compulsive behavior progressed as she aged.

---

50. Contemplating the caregiving experience, Patti Davis has recalled, "For a son or daughter to assume autonomy over a parent's life and say, 'I'm making the decisions now,' is a role reversal for which there is no preparation." "Behind Dianne Feinstein's Headlines Lies Another, Untold Story," *New York Times*, September 1, 2023.

2. Physical: Her stroke left her with diminished core strength, and her broken hip and subsequent surgical repair rendered her immobile.

3. Verbal: Although my mother retained her wit, she lost articulation—a problem I attributed to her aging throat and the insertion of a breathing tube during hip surgery. In time, I became the only one who could—or was patient enough to—understand her slurred words.

. . .

Because my mom's last years were spent in six different long-term care facilities, we experienced a range of hospice involvement. In her second home (where her hospice care began), the assisted facility nurse cultivated a relationship with hospice staff, promoted my mother's participation, and retained control over hospice supplies and equipment. During my mother's stay at her third residence, several hospice agencies (both for-profit and nonprofit) were present for various patients, and the facility's staff seemed less directly involved.

When the staff level decreased at my mother's third home, I asked for and received additional hospice help with bedtime transfers and toileting—for what seemed to be a maximum allotment of two evenings a week. The supplemental help—in fact, the same capable personnel—continued to appear twice weekly when my mother moved to her fourth place.

As cynical as I remained about hospice's overall presence, my mother continued to be more dependent, and I welcomed additional hands-on assistance. Beyond everything else, the word *hospice* was enmeshed in my understanding with the specific, sensitive moments of passage from life to death.

. . .

About six months into our hospice experience, a new social worker appeared on my mother's care team. Noticeably attentive and outgoing, she invited me to meet for lunch outside the facility. Welcoming a break, I chose a nearby restaurant that I'd visited many times.

Later, I read in my mother's notes that *I had requested* the lunch for emotional support with burnout, caretaking, and issues with the facility. We talked about my family history and my support network. The hospice writer said she "provided active and reflective listening, supportive counsel and validation of thoughts and feelings." What I remember most about our lunch meeting was that the social worker refused to eat. She apparently did a lot of *active* listening, and I passed her coping test. We never met outside of the facility again.

After two weeks, a note started to appear in my mother's record on the topic of family spiritual issues: Apparently, I'd reported talking to staff at Jewish Social Services for support, as well as other friends and Al-Anon, and I still worked out. In truth, I hadn't attended an Al-Anon meeting in a decade, but I was still working out five days a week, in an early-morning session for women over age forty who were affiliated with the university where I'd attended graduate school. And so, I'd become an intimate part of my mother's health record.

• • •

At various times during my mother's hospice experience, she was visited by less familiar nurses, who apparently certified the likelihood of her dying within six months. Because she wasn't suffering from a terminal illness, like cancer, a heart condition, or Alzheimer's disease, her general failing wasn't compatible with a calculable life span.

On January 18, 2017, our lead hospice nurse notified us of a meeting scheduled for the following afternoon. Familiar with care conferences that had occurred since my mom's initial days in assisted living, I assumed there'd be a roundtable discussion of issues that comprised her days: diet, activities, and incontinence. I expected to receive a follow-up report with a plan to make as-needed changes to medications and daily routine.

Following the familiar script, the care conference included the hospice social worker and nurse, but now we were joined by an additional hospice nurse (who'd completed a recent assessment of my mom's physical and mental status), as well as the head nurse from the memory care section, where my mother was being housed.

I brought my mother because the meeting was about *her*, and otherwise she'd wonder where I was. Besides, she sometimes voiced concerns of her own; and, even if she dozed, she remained a pleasant addition to any gathering. (At her former residence, she'd surprised the professionals who were discussing the facility's "no caffeine" policy by telling everyone in the room that she'd just read in *The New York Times* that coffee might add time to your life.)

As soon as we arranged our chairs—including my mom's wheelchair—around the conference table, the lead hospice nurse told me that my mom no longer qualified for services and would be discharged from hospice care.

● ● ●

Apparently, a face-to-face interview, required for each ninety-day service period, indicated that my mother wasn't dying quickly enough. I hadn't paid attention to the hospice clock that started ticking in 2015 (eighteen months earlier), and I hadn't focused on previous evaluations, during which my mother had apparently met the Medicare criteria:

Things to know

Only your hospice doctor and your regular doctor (if you have one) can certify that you're terminally ill and have a life expectancy of 6 months or less. After 6 months, you can continue to get hospice care as long as the hospice medical director or hospice doctor recertifies (at a face-to-face meeting) that you're still terminally ill.[51]

Only two months earlier, the hospice physician had attested that even though my mom had had a long length of stay on hospice, she remained eligible, with a trajectory of decline indicative of a six month or less life-expectancy.

Somehow, my mother had deviated from a normal course toward death. The transitional moment may have occurred two weeks before the care meeting, when she was observed as being pleasant and cooperative. My mom may have appeared too pleasant to die, and now her hospice care was being eliminated!

I wondered what time of day the evaluation had occurred, and, indeed, the previous face-to-face encounter was at 1:09 P.M. on January 10, 2017. My mother had just finished lunch and was likely to have been communicative and content.

● ● ●

Unfortunately, my mom's late-afternoon and evening anxieties had been intensifying for months. Eleven days earlier, she'd been verbally and physically aggressive towards the CNA performing our evening hospice assistance. Yelling and kicking people away, she did not calm down, even by the end of the visit. On that night, I'd called the hospice 24-hour line to apologize for my mom's behavior towards the CNA.

I was trying to maintain a cooperative care environment for my mom and me, but I had no idea that medical professionals had already initiated their plan for our removal from hospice. The care personnel assembled at the conference told me there was no opportunity to respond directly to the hospice determination, but if I

---

51. www.medicare.gov.

chose, I could appeal to a third-party arbitrator. Confused and frightened, I scribbled down the 800 number through which I could start an appeal.

• • •

Then the meeting topic switched to the wheelchair. I looked up and said, "Is this all about a wheelchair?" Indeed, the one piece of equipment my mom couldn't forfeit was a wheelchair—a standard Medicare-funded benefit of hospice life. I started to calculate how many steps backward we'd have to take: My mother's entire routine would change, from showering to emergency care visits, and I'd become responsible for ordering and purchasing medications, bandages, and sanitary and incontinence supplies. I had no idea how I'd select a wheelchair without transferring her to my car and driving to a medical-supply store to determine a proper fit.

I was exhausted. The assisted living facility was understaffed, and we depended on bedtime hospice assistance. I was also angry. The hospice nurse made note of my saying we were being "dumped"—and we were. We were being dumped by an irrational system of Medicare reimbursements, and, unfortunately, my frustration erupted in a conference room filled with caregivers who were neither responsible for the system nor capable of redesigning it.

• • •

A week earlier, my mother had been reported as needing total feeding assistance. The assisted living facility's scale had been broken, but was now working correctly, and her weight was recorded at 102.2 pounds. My mom, whose lifetime weight hovered between 130 and 135 pounds, was losing weight and suffering from irreversible vascular dementia, but her physical decline was not rapid enough to satisfy Medicare protocols for hospice eligibility. The final and, apparently, pivotal evaluation said she was "pleasantly confused throughout visit and able to answer simple questions."

My mother was found crawling on the floor attempting to get to the bathroom three days after that final assessment, but the decision to discharge her from hospice had already been made. The critical certification report denied any significant weight loss, changes in vocabulary, or med adjustments for several months. Anti-seizure medication was credited with preventing her seizures. She was noted to have bouts of loose stools and agitation, but both were "fairly well managed" with her current regimen.

The facts were that my mom—at 102 pounds—could not lose any more weight, and her speech was so slurred that my daughter and I were the only people patient enough to understand and anticipate her needs. The presenting diagnosis had not changed: My mother had endured one major stroke incident and a series of ministrokes at predictable intervals (usually every six weeks). For months, she'd been recorded as sleeping sixteen to eighteen hours a day. Since the previous summer, when I was asked to purchase over-the-counter medicine at an all-night pharmacy, I'd been secretly holding and dispensing supplemental doses of antidiarrhea medication.

My mom's agitation had led to falls and lacerations. A debilitating cough that one caregiver referred to as "fits" was unmanageable by cough medicines, pulverized pills, diet restrictions, or nebulizers.

Neither the professional staff assembled at the discharge meeting nor I possessed sufficient data or diagnostic information to predict a rate of decline. My mom lived for another fifteen months and often required nursing attention beyond the three hours a week allowed by the state in any assisted living facility. And now we were losing the supplemental hospice care for which we'd been encouraged to enroll.

• • •

In the contentious atmosphere of the care meeting, my mind drifted to the close bond between the Hollywood stars Debbie Reynolds and Carrie Fisher (mother and daughter), who, a month earlier, had died one day apart. I didn't realize how much their tragic, entwined life stories affected me until I said, "We're responsible for each other, Lillian and I . . . just like Debbie Reynolds and Carrie Fisher." I watched the lead hospice nurse write a note on her legal pad, and said, "I saw which part of my reactions you documented." Impacted by my mother's illnesses and her deteriorating quality of existence, I'd become almost as needy as she was. And in many ways, I was as deserving of supportive services.

I initiated an appeal as soon as the meeting ended. The process was straightforward, but working with an intermediary via an 800 number was fraught with delays, intermittent phone reception, and misunderstanding. I persisted until I was told I'd successfully filed a claim for continued Medicare-funded hospice coverage. But we had to wait seventy-two hours for a decision, and the weekend was coming up. I didn't know where, how, or whether to replace my mother's wheelchair. I didn't know when to leave my mom alone to purchase supplies, and I cried.

• • •

The following day, January 20, 2017, was Inauguration Day. Exactly eight years earlier, I'd sat next to my mother in the common area of her independent living complex. She and her friends, along with their families and other community members, assembled to watch history unfold on a big screen—the inauguration of the nation's first Black president. We'd been beyond excited, and I was more than grateful to witness the swearing-in with a politically engaged mom who'd been born two years before women won the right to vote.

Now, in 2017, the nation waited in disbelief. My mom knew what was happening, but she was not capable of communicating her understanding. Still, as the controversial day unfolded, I cherished the historic memory I could create—both with and for her.

As soon as the new president began to speak, I received a call from the hospice social worker. She didn't recant the decision or offer help with my mom's impending status change. She said, "Are you okay?" I said, "No, how can I be?" Her meeting notes had reported that I'd made a statement that implied consideration of harming myself and/or my mother.

I figured someone had misinterpreted my Carrie Fisher–Debbie Reynolds remark. Although I'd uttered it in a moment of love and concern, it was interpreted as a threat. In truth, neither Debbie Reynolds nor her daughter, Carrie Fisher, had harmed anyone! I told the social worker I wanted to watch the inauguration speech with my mom. She insisted that I call her back, and although I agreed, she reported that I hung up on her.

After the ceremony, I wheeled my mom to her usual table and began helping her access her food, as I did for most meals. I noticed the director of the long-term care complex enter the dining room and look around. He walked toward me and said we had to talk—immediately.

I said, "I want to continue helping my mother," but he said, "No." He led me to a nearby nurse's office, where I was stunned to see a police officer. I suspected (correctly) that the hospice agency had initiated a suicide watch—and I knew I had to remain calm.

The police officer's name was Amy. I made a quick connection, telling her that was my daughter's name. Then she asked me how I was feeling. I said I was experiencing emotional stress over the decision to curtail hospice help, and I acknowledged that I had not called the hospice social worker immediately after the televised swearing-in, because I'd planned to wait until my mom's lunch was over.

Officer Amy asked me again how I was feeling. I said, "Look, if anyone is concerned about how I'm taking care of myself, I just traded my precious VW Beetle for a four-wheel-drive SUV. My mother has never been this far from my house, and I know I'll need a safer car as soon as the roads become icy." I tried to speak very slowly and looked directly into her eyes. Amy must have determined I wasn't a threat to myself—or to anyone. She told me to go back to help my mother, and I did.

● ● ●

Over the next few days, three events occurred that prevented hospice from discontinuing services:

1. Even though the discharge notes read "no seizure since starting anti-seizure medication," my mother suffered her first ministroke in three months. She was immobile and nonresponsive for twenty-four hours. (I spent the night sleeping on her floor.)
2. The hospice physician recanted. He reported that my mother was terminally ill with a life expectancy of six months or less, and he acknowledged that she was debilitated with recurring seizures.
3. The third-party arbitrator informed me that the hospice organization staff either failed or neglected to submit the required termination documents.

● ● ●

Although my mother had suffered a seizure, as if on cue, we remained in a hospice conundrum: She was approaching the end of her life and required almost constant attention, but she was not declining at a calculable pace. My mom was not suffering from a standard hospice diagnosis for which Medicare could project that a death would occur within six months.

My mom was wheelchair-bound, had sustained a major stroke, and presented with ministrokes ("seizures") for which only I seemed to be keeping a record—and we both needed assistance. After each ministroke, she was weaker and more lethargic, and she required two people for every transfer. She needed me (or someone) to feed her, especially at the end of her meals. I'd been trying to weather the caregiving inconsistencies and staffing deficiencies of assisted living facilities, and now, as the end approached, I had to anticipate a collapse of major support: The cessation of Medicare/hospice involvement might occur at any time.

● ● ●

Since my comment about the dual tragedies of the codependent Hollywood mother and daughter, and despite the facts that Carrie Fisher had suffered from drug addiction and Debbie Reynolds had died from a stroke, my mother's file now gratuitously reported, that I had made suicidal statements.

The allegation was unfounded, but I knew I couldn't expend energy on correcting or expunging the record. (It wasn't *my* record.) My role was defined not by a callous, stigmatizing assessment, but by an eight-word sentence included in my mother's care file since her transfer to her third assisted living facility, nine months earlier: "Daughter Judy visits frequently to help reduce anxiety."

● ● ●

After three months went by, a different hospice physician reported on my mother and said her increasing weakness had resulted in five falls. Also, she was sleeping more during the day. Three months later, her decline was declared evident from a six-pound weight loss, coughing episodes, an episode of unresponsiveness, and ongoing falls. (One fall resulted in an ER visit for sutures in her right knee.) Once again, she was certified to have a life expectancy of six months or less.

What would become my mother's final six-month Medicare/hospice certification occurred in late July 2017. There'd been an increase in seizure activity, requiring medical intervention, and increased fatigue, resulting in longer sleeping hours. My mom was now coughing during meals and had a high risk for aspiration. Her recorded weight ranged between 98 and 102 pounds. On August 20, I reported she was sleeping all the time. She'd slept through her breakfast and through the previous three lunches. Her estimated life projection remained less than six months.

Nevertheless, her eligibility for hospice care was uncertain. On September 12, 2017, the hospice physician, social worker, compliance person, and home-care director met to review her case. On September 14, less than two months after the most recent evaluation and hospice extension, the hospice case manager recorded a reversal of medical opinion: My mother was no longer eligible for hospice services. She had vascular dementia, but because she could "converse, hold her head, and support her body trunk," her condition had been determined to have improved.

. . .

When a hospice social worker notified me on the morning of September 20, 2017, that (for the second time) my 99.5-year-old mother was not dying fast enough, we were in a more precarious position than we had been the previous January. I responded, "That's not acceptable. You know I can appeal, right?" and I added, "I guess I'll just tell my mom to have another seizure."

At 3:15 P.M., hospice left a message with my mother's PCP about the pending discharge due to failing hospice's eligibility criteria. Forty-five minutes later, the assisted living facility's owner and the director both told me my mother could not remain a resident in their facility without hospice involvement.

By then, advanced age, progressing dementia, and the appearance of the antipsychotic Haldol on her medications list made my

mom a risky and unwelcome long-term care occupant almost any-
where in the county, and we were far from retail services where I
might conveniently purchase supplies—including a new wheelchair. A hospice CNA noted that I was *very stressed out* about losing
hospice.

● ● ●

My mother's second discharge summary from hospice care
recorded her 10 percent weight loss over the previous six months
(from a high of 115 pounds to a current low of 96) as "slightly
underweight"). Her "agitation" was determined to be well
managed—yet she was reported to bite a caregiver on the arm, four
days later. The decisive review referred to only one "as needed"
dose of Haldol on September 1. In fact, she was receiving the
antipsychotic med three times a day. Ignoring the cough and
phlegmy expectoration, which had plagued her for more than a
year and would bring an end to her life eight months later, the
report said she did not have any symptoms that needed to
be managed. All symptoms were allegedly controlled with either
medications or current interventions, and, notably, she did not
have dysphagia leading to aspiration. (Actually, my mother had a
coughing spell at almost every meal and frequently couldn't continue eating.)

Most egregiously, the discharge note alleged that my mom's
seizures were managed because one hadn't occurred for three
months. But no one had asked for the record I'd kept for more than
five years—since before her major stroke. Even with medication,
my mother would continue to have sporadic ministrokes until her
final hospitalization, five months later.

● ● ●

Once again, I appealed to a third party. This time, my appeal was
denied. The decision was that the determination of the provider,

to terminate continued coverage of hospice services for my mother, was medically appropriate.

On September 27, 2017, my mother's lead hospice nurse at her fourth assisted living facility reported that her patient, who was approaching one hundred years of age, was "No longer terminally ill." Twenty-four hours later, my mom's hospice status changed to palliative care consult. Hospice nurses stopped visiting, and we proceeded on our own.

* * *

Five years after my mother died, the Sidney Hillman Foundation awarded *ProPublica* reporter Ava Kofman with the 2023 Hillman Prize for Journalism. Kofman's investigative work disclosed moral failings in hospice, an industry that has long been revered and misunderstood:

> . . . under the current system, as the number of patients with ambiguous prognoses rises, providers . . . are under financial pressure to abandon those who don't die quickly enough. It's a typically American failure of imagination that people with dire but unpredictable declines are all but left for dead.[52]

In the fall of 2017, a flawed, immoral Medicare-hospice nexus abandoned my needy mom.

* * *

Once hospice was gone, all prescriptions were transferred, and medications began to be ordered through a local pharmacy near the fifth assisted living site. Starting July 28, 2016 (seventeen months

---

52. Ava Kofman, "Endgame: How the Visionary Hospice Movement Became a For-Profit Hustler," *ProPublica* (copublished with *The New Yorker*), November 28, 2022.

earlier), my mother's hospice instructions were to verify expiration dates for comfort pack medications (including morphine) and to reorder yearly. The comfort pack was to be available in her assisted living facilities at all times, and the contents were to be used following the instructions of the hospice nurse. Now, possibly because of the absence of hospice oversight, a "cancel "message was sent to the pharmacy. In the autumn of my mom's life, morphine was discontinued, and I was not aware of the cancel message, the rationale, or the grave implications of proceeding without it.

· · ·

On October 4, after locating a new home, a wheelchair that was narrow enough for her slight frame, a shower chair, a raised toilet seat, a variety of over-the-counter medications, bandages, and sanitary supplies, I drove my exhausted mother to her fifth facility.

Taking advantage of a warm fall morning, I left my passenger asleep in the front seat of my vehicle while movers carried furniture, clothes, and boxes of belongings into her new space. I noticed the hospice physician who'd attended the termination meeting two weeks before and had not been willing to extend hospice coverage to a depleted woman. He was seated prominently, in the center of the common area of my mother's new home. He was attending to another issue and, clearly, not expecting to see me, either.

In the pre-COVID-19 era, the state required only a TB test and flu shot before an admission or transfer to a new assisted living facility. The hospice organization refused to initiate or read the TB test because the patient was no longer enrolled in services, so the assisted living director invited other residents to join us for the short private bus trip to a local clinic, where my mom could be immunized and billed through her private insurance.

Hospice continued to call about returning the Medicare-funded wheelchair. As soon as our new one arrived from Amazon and I'd assembled it, I scheduled a pickup.

• • •

Between April 7, 2015, and July 25, 2017, my mother had been certified fourteen times, by five different hospice physicians, for benefit periods lasting either two or three months—totaling over 850 days. Each certification predicted a death within six months. (In the spring of 2018, she was recertified for what would be one month—her last.)

In the meantime (from 2015 to 2018), Medicare spending on hospice providers in the United States rose from $15.9 billion to $19.6 billion—a 20 percent increase. Medicare beneficiaries of hospice services rose 12.3 percent—from 1.38 million to 1.55 million. The average length of stay rose almost 7 percent, from 86.7 days in 2015 to 92.6 days in 2019, while the average length of stay in an assisted living facility rose from 152 (in 2015) to 155 (in 2018).[53]

Although too late for my mom, health-policy experts are finally recognizing that the rigid six-month rule begs to be modified for dementia patients:

> Without a change in the six-month rule . . . many end-of-life care experts say Medicare should come up with a new rule to provide palliative care for people with dementia that focuses on pain and other quality of life issues, and that is tailored to the person's needs

---

53. *Hospice Facts and Figures,* 2021 ed. (Alexandria, VA: National Hospice and Palliative Care Organization), www.nhpco.org /factsfigures.

earlier in their illness. More intensive hospice services would be added later.[54]

In addition, long-term care observers have begun to focus on the business equation:

> Hospice programs with too many patients receiving care for more than six months raise some flags for Medicare, and are sometimes audited as a result—an expensive time-intensive process. If an audit uncovers seemingly inappropriate use of the benefit, the hospice might have to repay money that Medicare reimbursed, which can run up to millions of dollars.[55]

More than likely, the local hospice organization did not want to risk being audited on my mother's behalf.

Regrettably, the Medicare/hospice dilemma didn't resolve within my mom's lifetime. The percentage of patients discharged because they are no longer terminally ill hovers around 6.5 percent.[56] My mother was one such patient.

During the autumn of 2017 and early winter of 2018, the physician who oversaw my mother's dismissal from hospice visited her two times. Despite her additional ministrokes, intensified sundowning, and a fall from a toilet that required ER attention, he continued to deny her eligibility for care.

Recently, a health reporter wrote that "the greatest risk factor for the most common form of . . . late-onset Alzheimer's . . . is simply getting older. Above age 85 it affects a third of adults."[57] By

---

54. Emily Harris, "For End-Stage Dementia, Medicare Can Make Hospice Harder to Access," *Washington Post*, March 26, 2022.

55. Ibid.

56. *Hospice Facts and Figures*, 2021 ed. (Alexandria, VA: National Hospice and Palliative Care Organization), www.nhpco.org/factsfigures.

57. Dawn MacKeen, "Worrying if Alzheimer's Will Arrive," *New York Times*, August 16, 2022.

2019, a year after my mother died, the number of days spent as hospice recipients by patients with Alzheimer's, dementia, and Parkinson's exceeded the number of days for any other diagnosis (cancer, heart disease, stroke, or lung disease and pneumonia).[58] My mom remained more highly performing than a person diagnosed with Alzheimer's disease. The frequency of her seizures seemed to decline with certain medications, but her advanced age was an indication of her ever-shorter life span.

● ● ●

Four and a half centuries earlier, a French philosopher wrote:

> To die of old age is a death rare, extraordinary, and singular, and therefore so much less natural than the others: it is the last and most extreme sort of dying—and the more remote, the less to be hoped for. It is indeed the boundary of life beyond which we are not to pass, which the law of nature has pitched for a limit not to be exceeded; but it is withal a privilege she is rarely seen to give us to last till then. It is a lease she only signs by particular favor, and maybe to one only in the space of two or three ages, and then with a pass to boot, to carry him through all the traverses and difficulties she has strewed in the way of this long career. And therefore my opinion is that when once forty years old, we should consider it as an age to which very few arrive, for seeing that men do not usually proceed so far, it is a sign that we are pretty well advanced, and since we have exceeded the ordinary bounds which make the just measure of life, we ought not to expect to go much further. Having escaped so many precipices of death, whereinto we have seen so many other men fall, we should acknowledge that so extraordinary a fortune as that which has hitherto rescued us from

---

58. *Hospice Facts and Figures*, 2021 ed. (Alexandria, VA: National Hospice and Palliative Care Organization), www.nhpco.org/factsfigures.

those imminent perils—and kept us alive beyond the ordinary term
of living—is not likely to continue long.[59]

● ● ●

Six months elapsed between the cessation of my mother's hospice
eligibility and her readmission. By then, she'd spent eleven days
as a hospital inpatient, and she'd been transferred by ambulance
to her sixth assisted living facility. While withering from vascular
dementia, my mom was being irreversibly and almost uncontrol-
lably compromised by a medical condition that had been observed
twelve years earlier but had never before been included in her
hospice-related diagnosis: aspiration pneumonia.

The trigger words for hospice reacceptance were: "primary
diagnosis of senile degeneration of the brain and with secondary
diagnoses of dysphagia with aspiration pneumonia." One of the
days that lay ahead had now become her calculable life's end point,
and we could not expect to go further.

Within weeks, throat and swallowing complications brought
an uncomfortable end to life.

Although my mother was a reinstated recipient of hospice
services and a resident of a highly regarded assisted living facility, no gentle person or service assisted us on April 11–12, 2018,
the night of her passing. "Hospice," from the Latin word *hospes,*
encompasses dual concepts: health and hospitality. Sadly, for my
mother, in an almost three-year course as a hospice patient, neither goal was met.

---

59. Michel de Montaigne, "Of Age," c. 1576.

End of Life

On February 21, 2018, my mother and I visited her geriatric clinic for what would be the last time. My mom was stable: Her blood pressure was 136/75. Her temperature was 97 degrees Fahrenheit. Her pulse rate was 83, her oxygen saturation was 95 percent, and her respiration rate was 16. Her centennial birthday was just two months away. Happy when she saw her doctor's familiar face, my mom complimented him on his choice of shirt. When he told her his girlfriend had bought it for him, she giggled at the thought that she might soon attend a wedding (his). As my mom remembered later, "We all shared a good laugh."

The attendant at the appointment desk scheduled a return visit for an afternoon in the third week of August. Unknown then (but clearly possible), my mother would soon meet the Medicare requirement for hospice care: Her life expectancy was six months or less. By the time the August appointment arrived, my mom had died, and her remains were safely returned to the Florida sun—eternally tucked next to my dad's.

• • •

Because she was no longer a hospice patient, my mother wasn't entitled to Medicare-covered transportation. When I contemplated the snow-covered streets that would make it difficult for me to navigate the approach to the clinic, I hired a commercial van. I sat in the passenger seat, and my mom and her wheelchair were loaded into the rear. As healthy as she appeared, she grew tired and cranky on the return trip. Bouncing through fourteen miles of a rural road on our approach to her fifth assisted living facility, she repeatedly asked, "When will this be over?" Exhausted myself, I said, "We're almost there."

My mother's after-visit summary noted two concerns: For the past few weeks, she'd displayed stage-one ulcers on her lower back. I'd reported the lesions to her clinic, and we'd begun treating them. I wondered if they'd been irritated during the hours her bony, slouched body was supported by the base of her spine on the synthetic fabric of the oversize lounge chairs in the assisted living facility's common area. Although my mom appeared comfortable and protected in the same seating as her coresidents, and we'd achieved our goal of freeing her from the constraining wheelchair for extended periods of time, there might have been an unintended consequence: bedsores. The doctor recommended a barrier cream and a dressing. His notes read: "The most important thing is relief of pressure."

• • •

Then there was the cough: The woman who approached one hundred years old without suffering from cancer, diabetes, or a heart condition was destined to die from complications of a cough. She'd suffered from vomit-producing coughing spasms for over a year and a half. Nurses, the hospice physician (when he was still available), our family members, other residents' family members, and even other residents had all offered suggestions. My mom's pills were crushed into fine powder and administered in applesauce, and we'd limited dairy products. Still, her cough persisted.

Seven months earlier, the staff at her third assisted living home had stated "nothing more than usual." Hospice notes described the cough as "intermittent," but the sporadic timing rendered it no less consequential. For my aging mom, the unpredictable, debilitating spasms were taxing. Afraid and confused by the sudden onset, she looked at me and said, "I cannot help this," and I continued to seek a remedy.

Thinking that some foods might be difficult to swallow and digest, I shopped almost daily for nondairy milk and ice cream. We encouraged my mom to remain upright after meals, and we experimented with cough suppressants, inhalers, and nebulizers. The attacks were noisy and messy; for my mom, they were embarrassing. One nurse referred to them as "coughing fits." A hospice note stated that she'd been refusing her meds and spitting them out, even after the staff placed them in ice cream "like the family wishes." I was with her almost constantly, and I knew my mother wasn't refusing meds; she simply couldn't hold them down.

My mom was fastidious about her appearance. Before being confined to a wheelchair, she often left the table to wash spots off her clothing, even in restaurants and in the dining room when she was in independent living. Now, to help her retain her dignity, I purchased dozens of adult-size terry-cloth bibs, which helped fill the laundry bags of dirty clothing that I took home each night.

In his postvisit notes on February 21, 2018, the PCP wrote, "For the cough: Delsym is probably the most effective treatment we have currently." Indeed, I'd already become a frequent Delsym buyer at several Walgreens locations.

* * *

One day later, as I was helping prepare my mom for bed, I was startled by the deepest cough I'd ever heard—a low, almost inhuman roar. She repeated the guttural tones over the next thirty-six hours. The gruff, loud tone didn't seem to hurt her, but I became frightened. I thought eating—even small snacks—might be the cause. Suddenly, we were faced with a new situation, and we were wandering through strange, unfamiliar territory.

Attempting a long shot, I called the physician who still hadn't recertified my mom for hospice care. When he'd dismissed her, five months earlier, he said he'd be available for dementia symptom management, as well as medication management, thru the palliative care program (which I never understood). Since that time, the physician had participated in one visit to adjust the dosage and timing of the antianxiety medication lorazepam, and then a second polite but informal visit six weeks later.

Seventeen days before the onset of the roaring cough, I'd requested a medical records review, preliminary to readmitting my mother to hospice. The hospice physician had responded that she was still not eligible for enrollment. He said if she experienced repeated seizures and more profound lethargy, or lost weight, or had another new pattern of decline, she would be *likely* to become eligible. In fact, in the four months since her hospice dismissal, my beleagured mother had experienced two ministrokes and a fall from the toilet, the latter resulting in a lost tooth, a forehead laceration, and a trip to an ER.

● ● ●

Regrettably, I miscalculated the chances of an appeal that was based on a new, strange cough. The doctor told me a cough was not within my mom's accepted hospice diagnosis, and he said he couldn't visit her because just that week he'd had plastic surgery on his eye. He told me to contact her PCP, and he scheduled his return visit for March 9, 2018. By then, my mother would be a hospital inpatient, suffering from life-ending symptoms, and I'd be trying to locate another assisted living facility (her sixth), where she would die.

The next day, I drove my weakened mother—this time, as a frail passenger in my own car—to the emergency room. After several hours, the staff decided to refer her for a swallow test, which they couldn't schedule until the next morning. The nurses assumed I'd stay overnight and moved two beds into a room adjacent to the ER suite—a large room that routinely held one oversized bed. With more attention than my mother had been accustomed to in that hospital, we became overnight occupants of the bariatric suite.

When morning arrived, the nurse on duty refused to let me help transfer my mother to a wheelchair in the manner to which she'd become accustomed—with the simple pivot disc we'd used for four years. Over the next few days, I watched anxiously as caregivers shifted my limp mother from stiff chairs and unceremoniously placed her onto her bed. My mom, holding her chest and belly, told them, "You're hurting me." Looking back, I wonder at what painful moment she lost the physical strength and muscle memory to participate in transfers.

◦ ◦ ◦

My mother was no longer being consulted about her own body. She was lifted back and forth like a rag doll. More than anything, she was confused by the bedside commode. She could see into the en suite bathroom and pointed to a familiar porcelain toilet. She knew she wasn't being understood and tried the simplest words: "I want the wood." What she meant was that the floor surrounding the toilet in the bathroom was polished hardwood. She was being ignored, and she knew it.

Typical of a hospital unit, caregivers cycled through without time or patience to listen to a weakened patient. My mother regressed from verbally responsive to garbled speech to displays of physical aggression, trying to hit and bite the hospital staff.

Adding to our discomfort, the report on the swallow test was inconclusive. The nurses told me, "Something showed up," but because hospital orders weren't followed, and my mom was delivered to the testing room in the wrong wheelchair, they weren't able to tilt her aging frame back far enough to retrieve clear images. I never understand what X-ray technicians point out on their computer screens, and this learning opportunity was no exception. I was at a low point, exhausted from confusion, concern, and lack of sleep. When the hospital staff tried to describe my mother's problem, I saw only a gray-and-white blur on the monitor.

No matter what I heard over the next week and a half, while my physically and cognitively diminished mom lay in a crowded, noisy room, I processed our problem as *good woman with old throat.* No one asked me, but I thought her weakness could be attributed to a surgical procedure she'd undergone when she was ten years younger, after a diagnosis of aspiration pneumonia, or, perhaps, to the breathing tube that had been inserted during hip-repair surgery three years earlier.

I sensed that at this end-of-life stage, the issue wasn't *diagnosis,* but *prognosis,* although I was incapable of understanding what the hospitalist said to me. I asked him to communicate with my older daughter—and I don't think I heard what she said to me, either. Looking back, I know the doctor tried to deliver our options: We could continue to offer soft food and thickened liquid mixtures that would prolong my mother's life, or we could choose not to do so.[60]

---

60. On September 14, 2024, as this work was being readied for publication, Paula Span reported in the *New York Times* ("Three Medical Practices Older Patients Should Question") that a study from the Feinstein Institutes for Medical Research in Manhasset, NewYork, found that liquid thickening doesn't actually prevent aging patients from drawing liquids into their lungs and developing aspiration pneumonia.

• • •

On the night when a blizzard was forecast, the floor staff wheeled in a folding cot so that I could stay with my mother rather than drive home in the storm. My dog had been in the room that afternoon, and he remained through the snowy night. Added to corridor activity, the requisite medication schedule, and my mom's discomfort, my folding cot—merely a sharp bedspring poking up through a worn mattress—meant that no one slept.

The next afternoon, the kind owners from my mother's fifth residence visited, and one of them referred to my mom as being on her deathbed. Although my mother was failing—disheveled and withdrawn, with a light green bow in her hair—I was secretly insulted and refused to understand or accept that she was at the terminal stage. Day after day, the social worker came to ask me about our plans. The only message I processed was that we had to move my mom to her next (sixth) assisted living facility.

I will always wonder if or how my mother's life and comfort were weighed against the hospital's reputation. Four years later, *The New England Journal of Medicine* reported:

The Centers for Medicare and Medicaid Services (CMS) Hospital Value-Based Purchasing Program penalizes facilities with high 30-day mortality, which is counted from the date of admission. This penalty is a strong incentive to avoid hospitalizing patients for what may be a "terminal admission" because it could increase the hospital's death rate. Mortality also figures prominently in ranking systems used by both CMS and *U.S. News and World Report*. CMS excludes from ranking-related calculations patients who were enrolled in hospice at any time during the 12 months before the admission, including the first day of the admission, but *U.S. News and World Report* does not. Staff members who are unaware of exclusion rules may believe it's safer to avoid admitting patients who are near death—regardless of their hospice status—to preserve the hospital's reputation.[61]

The authors of the article proceeded to recommend that those with hospice involvement be excluded from death statistics.

We . . . suggest aligning all quality-measurement systems, especially the ratings of *U.S. News and World Report*, with CMS's system that excludes hospice patients from mortality reporting. This exclusion would need to be well publicized to avoid confusion.[62]

●　●　●

I thought about the autumn day, five years earlier, when I also asked the hospitalist at the same hospital to admit my mother. According to the ER record, "The patient and her mother elected to go home."

I'm not a trained diagnostician, but in September 2013, I knew that my mother had suffered or was suffering from a stroke. I had not "elected to go home." It was a Friday, and I had no instructions on how to care for her over the weekend. Frustrated and alone, we packed up and left. Four days later, my mom was admitted to a stroke unit at another hospital.

Now, we'd come full circle, and, once again, I had to organize my thoughts. As my mind cleared, I began to understand:

---

61. Melissa W. Wachterman, M.D., M.P.H., Elizabeth A. Luth, Ph.D., Robert S. Semco, B.S.E., and Joel S. Weissman, Ph.D., "Where Americans Die—Is There Really 'No Place Like Home'?" *New England Journal of Medicine* 386, no. 11(March 2022):1009.

62. Ibid.

1. The medical facility, where she'd been an inpatient for more than a week, had no intention of holding my mother until she died.

2. My mother was begging for water, but she could ingest only soft foods and thickened liquids.

3. How and what she ate would be my choice.

4. The social worker had one purpose: to help us move out.

5. No area skilled nursing facility would accept my mother, because she'd been prescribed a presumably threatening psychedelic drug—Haldol. Instead of viewing that fact as an indication that her emotional distress was being monitored and treated, the assisted living and nursing home community refused to admit her.

6. Hospice staff might show up to help process a transfer, but there were no hospice services in the hospital.

● ● ●

In the midst of the standoff, someone (the PCP, the hospital physicians, the hospice doctor, or the assisted living admissions teams) made the decision to change my mother's meds. Suddenly, she stopped taking Haldol and was given another antipsychotic, olanzapine. I'd given up interjecting myself into drug discussions, and I had no idea why one medication was unacceptable while the other was less threatening. (Mostly, I was relieved not to have to discuss the delay in my mom's hospital discharge any longer.)

The choices for the next home came down to two: an assisted living facility located eleven miles east, and another, over seven miles west. Only I could visit the sites, select a room, and begin the admissions process. Somehow, I accomplished the tasks while maintaining a nearly constant presence in the hospital room.

I made the lonely trip to the more distant place in vain. Although he hadn't mentioned limited capacity during our phone call, the director could only offer a double room.[63] As the next profoundly difficult month unfolded, I often wished my mother was in many other environments, but I allowed room configuration to be my guide. I chose her sixth assisted living facility because it offered a private room with a large bathroom and accessible shower.

* * *

On a chilly Monday morning, ambulance personnel appeared on the hospital floor to transfer my mom. Balancing white plastic bags stuffed with her personal belongings, I was asked to sign a release—in case the patient died along the way.

I had followed or met conveyances for ministrokes, a major stroke, lacerations, and falls. When she was able, my mother would chat with the "nice" attendants. Now, as the ambulance drivers wheeled her along the hospital corridor, one nurse looked at me and said, "You know you could have moved her last Friday." Up until the previous Friday, my mom was being medicated with the maligned drug Haldol. I made a mental note to report the remark— as I'd considered recording other incidents in online post-visit surveys—but I backed off because I was as relieved as anyone that we were leaving.

Depressed and tired, I wandered through several floors of seemingly identical vehicles and climbed indistinguishable concrete staircases until I found my blue SUV in the dimly lit parking

---

63. As I've become capable of extending a long view to the eldercare industry, I've come to suspect that I didn't mishear. The director was probably cautious about requests from overwrought family members who were trying to secure rooms for patients being dismissed from the nearby hospital—seeking beds in which to die. I viewed the unacceptable room because that's what he showed me once he met me.

structure. I inserted my visitor's pass into the familiar machine at the gate and proceeded along the same route as the ambulance. I was trailing my mother during her last hospital discharge.

We headed for a CCRC we'd visited twelve years before, when there'd been no vacancy in the independent living apartments. Author and law professor Daniel Jay Baum wrote:

> What happens to our parents on their final journey affects us, their adult children. One day we will be making the same journey. How we help our parents may shape how we respond when our children, our friends, or other relatives try to help us. One day most of us will make such choices, or they will be made for us. We travel in our parents' wake.[64]

* * *

My dying mother was reenrolled in hospice four hours after she arrived, and she began receiving the familiar level of visits from hospice nurses and a hospice social worker. Everything seemed to slow down and, apparently, I started to relax. Her notes described a "warm supportive family permitting expression of feelings." Spring had appeared, and a long, low window allowed rays of afternoon sun to shine in.

But the moves had taken their toll. My mom slept and often refused to eat or take her meds. Caregivers, who were usually confused by her slurred speech, noted that she said "Go to hell" when I tried to reattach the thin plastic oxygen tubing that had slipped from her nostrils.

My mother still thought if she raised her arm and hand (as she had in the common area of her fifth assisted living facility), someone would know she wanted to use the bathroom. When she thought she was being ignored, she resorted to the most effective

---

64. Daniel Jay Baum, *Assisted Living for Our Parents: A Son's Journey* (Indianapolis: iUniverse, Inc., 2011), p. 6.

means of communication she knew—kicking obstacles and people away and attempting to bite.

• • •

A wellness and parenting reporter, writing about toddlers' capacity to learn to self-regulate, said, "Being mad is a basic emotion, and learning to cope with it can make everyone's life easier."[65] My mother was at the end of her life, not the beginning, but her rage was as raw and uncontrolled as the children the reporter described: "when they went for it they *really* went for it: screaming, sobbing, full-body shaking—the works."[66]

One noted child and family psychologist recommends diversionary techniques for children, such as displaying pictures of other children smiling or laughing. "I like to say the best form of anger management is feeling understood. . . . Often when we're angry, underneath we feel scared, we feel misunderstood, and we feel disconnected."[67]

When my daughter flew from New York to spend her last week with her grandmother, she brought a stuffed doll with wide eyes, a permanent smile, and a yellow hair bow. My mother had lost the dexterity or interest to unbutton and unzip the doll's clothes, but she embraced the small body, smiled, and wondered what to name it—a welcome, calming diversion.

Unfortunately, my disconnected mother had long since entered the realm where her emotions were unwelcome and misunderstood. Her outbursts led to staff reliance on "as needed" anti-anxiety compounds—not anger-management techniques.

• • •

---

65. Catherine Pearson, "Kids Can Get Better at Handling Anger,"
    New York Times, July 12, 2022.
66. Ibid.
67. Jazmin McCoy, author of *The Ultimate Tantrum Guide,* quoted in Ibid.

A complex drug narrative had begun four and a half years before, when a hospitalist recorded a reaction to opioids: "Oxycodone Reaction: Dizziness, Multiple falls while on it." Because of that note, my mother's initial admission to hospice included mention of an "allergy" to oxycodone. When hospice ceased treating my mother, six months before her death, the end-of-life opioid (morphine) that had been included in her typical hospice comfort pack for more than a year was removed from her medications list. I remained unaware that, even upon readmission to hospice, morphine was never reordered.

Now, when my mother was terminal, a note from the hospice pharmacist documented my mother's *intolerance* to oxycodone: "Check to see if she has tolerated other opioids in the past as she may benefit from use of an opioid for treatment of pain or dyspnea as she approaches end of life." Despite the note, no one checked with me about opioid intolerance. To my knowledge, my mother had once reacted to oxycodone as any woman in her nineties would have: In her own words, she'd felt "drunk" from the dizziness. Preoccupied with patient mobility, comfort, and diet, I could no longer keep track of drugs, and the doctors no longer consulted me.

• • •

For the final time, I engaged in a discussion about transferring my mother via pivot disc—as we'd done before her hospital stay. The facility's intake person referred the decision to a PT consult. I attended the evaluation, and we demonstrated a basic transfer (from wheelchair to chair) to a therapist, who wasn't interested. What I recall was someone talking to me about exercises, which I knew were meaningless for my mom—she was beyond comprehending or participating in exercises.

I had to accept that the pivot disc was history, and we began to suffer the indignities of a battery-run Hoyer lift. Every transfer—to and from bed, to and from the wheelchair, or to and from the toilet—now required two caregivers plus a mechanical lift.

This was the procedure for my mom to be moved from her wheelchair to a toilet:

1. She was wrapped in a body sling.
2. She was hoisted from the wheelchair to the bed.
3. Her clothes (frequently soiled) were removed.
4. Naked from the waist down, she was placed back in the body sling, elevated, and swung to the toilet.

Something about the design of her corner bathroom, large though it was, made the transfer complicated: If the caregivers forgot to prop the door open, they had to abort the transfer, pull my mother aside (half naked and fully exposed), adjust the door, and begin again.

Safety regulations and common sense required two caregivers (although even one was often difficult to locate) for every transfer, so we waited and waited. I offered to help, but I was rebuffed. The fact that I'd assisted or accomplished her transfers since my mom broke her hip, three years earlier, made no difference. More than once, when the caregivers arrived, pushing a lift in front of them, they realized the battery pack required recharging, and we waited while they searched for a replacement.

I tried to show the caregivers that my mom could shift her body and cooperate, so they could remove her pull-up pants while she was still in the wheelchair. Perhaps they'd eliminate several steps in the intricate toileting process and save everybody's precious time and energy. But a toilet transfer was done only one way: from wheelchair to bed, *undress,* from bed to toilet, from toilet back to bed, *redress,* and, finally, from bed back to wheelchair.

A vision still haunts me from the spring morning when I walked into my mother's room and saw her splayed on the bed— stark naked. The Hoyer lift was there, and I could only assume the caregivers had been interrupted during the convoluted process, then forgotten or neglected to return. My mother, at ninety-nine years of age, was lying on her bed, uncovered, uncomfortable, and naked.

● ● ●

Over a decade before, following one of my mom's hospital visits, we'd agreed upon DNR status. The thought of her dying was remote, but a social worker encouraged us to sign by saying, "You don't want anyone pounding on her chest and breaking her ribs, do you?" I knew I didn't. Pounding on my mother's chest was beyond the range of comfort or necessity.

But one afternoon, during her recent hospital stay, I entered her room and witnessed a nurse pressing on my mom's chest and asking her to start breathing. I was speechless—too startled to intervene—and her breathing resumed. Time has passed, but I still wonder if I observed an unauthorized attempt to resuscitate. Maybe I was supposed to object, but I was exhausted, and my reaction time had decreased. Also, I recalled the hospitalist saying my mother couldn't die in that hospital.

From the day she was admitted to the hospital until the moment she died in assisted living, my mom was tethered to low-flow oxygen via a nasal tube. I was told the oxygen was for comfort, not for lifesaving resuscitation, and more than anything, I wanted her to be comfortable. But how was an emotionally overburdened, untrained daughter expected to oversee patient comfort?

When the mother of author and devoted son Dave Iverson was ninety-five years old and he was making decisions about care protocol, he asked the hospice nurse, "So why did some life-support treatments feel appropriate, and others not?" Iverson recalled:

> As we talked it through, the concept that would guide our decision-making became clearer: to provide comfort without prolonging life unduly. . . . Giving her extra oxygen through a non-invasive nasal tube would keep her comfortable if her breathing became more labored, but it wouldn't cure anything or prolong her life in a consequential way.[68]

While Iverson appears to have felt included in the discussion, I recall being *informed* that there would be oxygen. I knew my mother was troubled by the nose clip, which consistently fell to one side of her face. The long green cord that was sometimes attached to a noisy tank in her bathroom frequently tripped caregivers, who could only kick it away—and forget to reconnect it—as they toileted her via the cumbersome Hoyer lift.

● ● ●

Besides comfort and mobility, I remained anxious about diet. In her final month in assisted living facility number six, my mom tolerated being wheeled to a large room filled with round dining tables, where she slowly consumed limited amounts of thickened drinks and softened food. I knew she hoped for better meals and probably craved at least one more grilled cheese and tomato sandwich.

Because the efficient kitchen staff could provide a variety of thickened liquids, a colorful supply of fruit drinks and straws was stored along one wall. Nevertheless, ten days before I lost her, I interceded when an unfamiliar caregiver walked from the medication cart toward my mother with pills and a plastic cup of freshly

---

68. Dave Iverson, *Winter Stars* (Durham, NC: Light Messages Publishing, 2022), p. 190.

poured water. Because of her high aspiration risk, my mother was allowed *only* thickened liquids. The med passer either forgot or wasn't paying attention. In my heart, I knew our support was fading.

On Tuesday, April 3, I arrived during lunchtime. My mom was already in the dining area, and I could see she was slouched to her right. A stained bed pillow was stuffed beside her, to help hold her upright. Not thinking about anything but reaching her, I tied my dog along the side wall of the dining room.

Although others at the table were eating or appeared to have eaten lunch, no one had served food to my mom. The napkin at her place was still folded, the utensils were unused, and the drinking glass was empty. Her hands and the bed pillow were stained with something red, which I could only guess was from breakfast—maybe jelly. At 12:30, long after the usual serving time, I wheeled my unfed mom away.

I noticed the hospice nurse and social worker sitting in an alcove in the hall. I could barely explain how many things I thought were wrong in the dining room. The hospice nurse suggested we visit the facility's head nurse. My mother had been a resident for over two weeks, and I still didn't know the head nurse had an office—I'll accept responsibility for that oversight.

I told the head nurse I thought no one had cleaned my mom after breakfast. She was still reclining on a jelly-stained bed pillow that had been used to bolster her in the wheelchair, and her hands were sticky. I said my mother's setting contained no lunch plate, and her eating utensils and cup appeared untouched. Instead of a calming comment such as "How can we help you?" or even "Let's look into this," her response was, "How do you know?" I guess I *didn't*. Our entourage (mom, wheelchair, hospice nurse, social worker, little dog on leash, and I) returned to my mother's room and started cleaning her up.

The facility's social worker came into the room and asked, "Is hospice still working with you?" She said she wanted to talk to me. She directed me toward the door and told me the dog wasn't allowed in the dining room. That was all. I did not react well.

My mother never regained her sharp articulation after her hip surgery, three years before. She'd been prescribed sessions with a speech therapist, but she'd deemed the practice activities childish and refused to participate. As time went on, I became the sole person who was familiar enough with her reactions and desires to anticipate her needs and relay her garbled messages to caregivers. On that day, my mom looked up from the noisy discussion about neglecting her at breakfast (or lunch) and the errant dog, and she found her clear diction long enough to say, "Shut up, everyone!"

* * *

Despite my best intentions, communication with the staff of the sixth assisted living facility became strained. I felt as though we were perceived as transient, and they didn't appear to be working either with us or for us.

I have a short video of my mother telling me she knew she wasn't receiving good care. My overarching goals became patient safety and staff cooperation, and I tried to communicate my expectations with the hospice social worker. On the hospice 24-hour line, I left a message asking for an update on the interaction between my mom and her CNAs. I said I wanted us all to be on the same page on how to best approach my mom when she became combative.

Over several years, I'd built a relationship with the state's long-term care ombudsman. Since the time my mom lived in her first assisted living facility, the ombudsman had provided professional advice and respite. Now she suggested moderating a meeting between the assisted living nurses and me, and I thought that a moderated discussion could be a means of conflict resolution—surely, not a threat. I missed the ombudsman's visit, but she left her card—which must have been spotted and misinterpreted. The facility's record stated, "Judy has been threatening staff she is going to report to the state. She states the cares [*sic*] they are providing are incorrect and abuse [*sic*]."

Under stress, did I say that? Was I threatening? It seems to me that the opposite of *care* is *neglect,* and, except for the two incidents of a sexual advance to my mom and a badly injured arm, I did not have the authority or ability to attribute *abuse* to any action—or inaction.

Even if I had time to prepare an official complaint or submit a report on any issue, my effect would have been minimal. A journalist whose mother was evicted from an assisted living home has pointed out:

> Wisconsin runs a Provider Search database on actions involving nursing homes and other long-term care facilities, but its functionality is minimal. There is currently no way to do searches by category of offenses or to obtain other aggregate information . . . [the state's complaint tracking website] is in need of substantial improvement.[69]

In previous facilities, I'd submitted email complaints to relevant agencies about the lack of caregivers (especially in the evenings), inadequate food choices, uncooperative staff, and a deficient telephone system. Sometimes I received lengthy explanations or my comments were transferred to an agency round robin, but most of my concerns were deemed unsubstantiated. Now, the reality was that I had other things on my mind.

Within days, my mother stopped eating in the dining room. Her food was ordered from a printed menu and brought to her bedside. She lost either interest or capacity—or both—and her

---

69. Bill Lueders, "Evicting the Elderly: 'A Sad Thing That Happened,'" *The Progressive Magazine,* August 18, 2022.

consumption became almost infantile. Sometime over the weekend of April 7–8, she ceased all food intake, and her nurses stopped trying to dispense scheduled medications—even "mood/behavior" medications.

In a timeline that remains overshadowed by a daughter's enduring guilt, I'll never know if a prescription for oxycodone to address back pain triggered my mother's stroke. And I'll never know if the activities person at her second assisted living facility (who told me she found my mother on the floor) hurried into room 113 without knocking and, in her typical high-energy entrance, either startled or pushed my off-balance mom backward, precipitating a fall and a crippling hip fracture. Similarly, I don't know if one last coughing episode caused my mom to stop eating during a weekend in early April 2018.

On a meal receipt that remained on a food tray in her room, I read that (against medical orders) an uncut portion of salmon, asparagus, and nonthickened water were delivered for one of my mom's lunches. I wasn't there to assist with the feeding, and I have no idea if she ate even one bite. Ironically, the food choices were her lifelong favorites—and apparently, the time had come.

• • •

I should have been prepared for what would happen next. From initial days as a hospice patient, three years before she died, my mother's hospice records repeated the statement: "Patient/family supported in discussing and sharing feelings/concerns related to approaching death." Beginning in July 2015, hospice notes had become more detailed:

END OF LIFE EDUCATION
Determine Family Understanding of What to Expect
ENGAGE PATIENT/PCG [primary care giver] IN LIFE REVIEW
Educate Patient /PCG re Foods/Fluid at EOL

Educate re: End of Life
Educate to Contact [hospice] in Emergency
Give Pt/Family Opportunity to Talk about Death
Introduce Approaching Death Discussion

I'd participated in multiple stressful conversations about my mom not dying soon enough to continue receiving Medicare certification for hospice care. I'd listened and responded as the topic jumped from patient health decline to funeral homes and cremation—then, to self-care. I'd engaged with hospice staff several days a week for almost thirty-six months, but no one described life's last moments.

I was seventy-five years old, and I'd never witnessed a death. Nearly three years earlier, a jarring early-morning call erroneously and cruelly reported my mother's death, and I met with a hospice grief counselor. I'd worked with and befriended a succession of hospice nurses, and I visited and had lunch with a hospice social worker. At no time had any care personnel or instructions made me aware of the signs and sounds of distress—the loud struggle signaling the final moments of life.

So, I self-educated about the dying process. Every Wednesday morning for two years, I'd granted myself a leisurely breakfast with a friend whose mother was a resident of a different combination of area assisted living facilities. After a period of failing health, my friend's mother died, and as weeks passed, we began to discuss their final hours together. For the first time, I heard about the loud, labored breathing of the dying. My friend told me she could still replicate the deep sounds of her mother's last breaths.

• • •

On Sunday, April 8, 2018, a close friend visited my mom and another resident of the care facility. Her husband, a recently retired physician, accompanied her. We all sat with my mom, who was sleeping, as she always seemed to be, at this stage.

The physician/husband/friend asked me what my mother was doing in that place. Why hadn't she been transferred to the hospice inpatient facility? I had no answer. Possibly because of concerns about psychotropic meds, when we were struggling to find a place to house her after her recent hospital stay, the hospice complex was not considered to be an option.

When I posed the question to hospice staff later in the day, I was told my mother didn't have any symptoms that couldn't be managed where she was currently residing.

● ● ●

The days passed quietly. I played classical music through a Bluetooth receiver, and I waited for the sun to come through the bedroom window.

On April 8, my mother started fidgeting and twitching, seemingly uncomfortable in her own skin. I called to request a hospice visit and said I couldn't understand why the assisted living facility hadn't called to report my mother's condition: The hospice report said I had "multiple things" I was complaining about regarding my mom, including that she was uncomfortable. I didn't know I was complaining; I thought the hospice mission was to assure a *comfortable,* dignified ending of life.

On Tuesday, April 10, my mom allowed me to polish her nails. She had at least a dozen bottles of red polish, including duplicates of her lifelong preference, Revlon's Cherries in the Snow, which she chose. She saw her clean hands, and she liked them. A hospice caregiver, whom we'd not met before, stopped in and offered to massage my mom's dry skin with gentle lotion, and I relaxed with her.

Early in the afternoon of Wednesday, April 11, I realized that my mother had a fever. I called hospice and, after an hour, a nurse arrived. By then, the fever had subsided, but I finally had an opportunity to ask about the loud breathing that my friend had described hearing just before *her* mother died.

"Oh, yes, you'll hear it," the nurse told me. Then he said, "She'll be breathing very loudly, and you'll hear her stop for a time. It's really important that you don't stop breathing then also. Keep on breathing . . . and wait. She'll start breathing again." Those were my instructions from hospice on death and dying: *Keep breathing. Do not stop. She'll start breathing again.*

The hospice nurse turned my mom over in the bed and went to see another patient. I could hear louder breaths, but I had no idea what *loud* meant. When the nurse walked by in the hallway, I asked him to come back for a minute. Was that the breathing we were anticipating? He said, "She just sounds different because I repositioned her." He said she was fine, and I should go home and try to sleep. I had no frame of reference, and I'm sure no one does in those moments. My mom was fine, he said, so I went home.

. . .

In my own living room, seven and a half miles away, I fell onto my sofa. I tried to keep reminding myself I hadn't eaten supper. In fact, I hadn't had any food since breakfast. At 9:33 P.M., I received a call from a nurse I'd met several days before, when he was in my mother's room. He said he was leaving soon. His shift was over at 11:00, but he thought my mother might not last until then.

I called my daughter, who'd spent a week at the end of February, supporting me, visiting her grandmother, and helping organize and clear the room at the previous assisted living facility. We stayed on the phone for the sixteen-minute ride west. The roads were clear, yet the city looked dark, empty, and oddly unfamiliar.

I wanted to reach my mom's room as soon as possible, but I was held up by the nighttime security system at the front door. I waited in the building's foyer, and I started to shiver.

• • •

When I saw my mother, a person I did not recognize (apparently, the night nurse) was wielding a square sponge on a stick, attempting to clear mucus from a partially open mouth. I asked if she had a bulb syringe, but she said she did not. Somehow, I remembered that the standing orders required "suction as needed to clear airway." Without calculating how the length of time was compressing, I said I'd leave to buy a syringe at Walgreens.

Of course, no drugstores were open. Awash in sadness, I observed the clumsy process and recalled how one novelist, the author of books on eldercare, wrote about her own dying mother: "She flinched under the stubby fingers of the . . . nurse. She was nothing but a sick old woman. Who cared what she thought?"[70]

• • •

My son in Denver called at 10:43 P.M. Over the phone, he could hear his grandmother's labored breathing and my conversations with the nurse. I asked why my mother was struggling and if there were meds that might grant relief. The nurse said, "Morphine has not been prescribed." I was beyond anger and shock. I knew the standard hospice comfort pack contained morphine and that there had to be an opiate available.

As a fallback, I asked about the drug lorazepam, which I knew was listed for anxiety and aggression on the medications list from the recent geriatric clinic visit. The nurse said she couldn't dispense more lorazepam because the orders read every four hours. I said, "The schedule is every three hours." While my mother lay on her deathbed, struggling to breathe, the professional caregiver in a licensed eldercare facility left the bedside, telling me she had to "work on clarifying" the lorazepam discrepancy.

---

70. Marina Lewycka, *A Short History of Tractors in Ukrainian* (New York: Penguin Books, 2005), p.6.

My mother and I were caught in the ultimate communications snafu, and I didn't have the authority to extricate us.[71] I knew lorazepam had been administered sometime within the previous four hours, but now, my good mother would continue her labored breathing until her last breath, with no intervention or assistance from opiate comfort meds.

• • •

Where and how had I lost track of the prescribed morphine? Was it even my responsibility? More than two years before, a nurse at the second assisted living facility reported "increased anxiety and decline in function." She also reported that she'd spoken with me, the daughter, and that I'd okayed comfort medications. A hospice nurse contacted my mother's PCP, requesting orders for an end-of-life comfort pack. After the nurse at the assisted living facility told me comfort pack medications were on board, I had no reason to doubt that morphine would be available when we needed it.

A year *before* my mother died, an unfamiliar CNA told me she'd administered morphine from the comfort pack because my mom had fallen from her bed and was complaining of nonspecific aches and pain. The results were that my mom remained lethargic most of the day.

My mother had been either sliding or tumbling onto a floor pad almost every other night. She needed closer observation and more immediate response to her bathroom alerts. The care staff

---

71. My mother's last two medications lists, recorded on April 8, 2018 (three days before her death) and April 12, 2018 (the reported day of her death), read: "Lorazepam (ATIVAN) 0.5 MG tab 30 tab Sig—Route: Take 1 tab by mouth every 3 hours as needed (agitation or anxiety. Hospice patient. Do not fill until requested by facility.)—Oral MORPHine [*sic*] 15 MG tab 30 tab Sig—Route. Take .05 tabs by mouth every 3 hours as needed for shortness of breath or pain (Hospice patient. Do not fill until requested by facility.)—Oral."

needed an understanding of the mechanics of *fall prevention*. The time would come when I would expect morphine to be accessible, but on a random morning, a year before her death, my mother hardly required a controlled opiate. Hospice provided teaching to the facility CNA and checked on my mom frequently. They reinforced not to give the comfort med, morphine:

> Morphine is there for EOL [end of life]. Patient has scheduled Tylenol and ibuprofen PRN [as needed]. Call hospice if patient has pain unmanaged with these medications.

. . .

Now, on an April night in 2018, the end-of-life need for morphine had arrived. My mother was fighting a descent toward her "long sleep," as she once called it, without any intervention or promise of relief. The night nurse told me I could climb into the narrow bed with her patient, but my mother's breathing was so labored, I didn't want to complicate the struggle. I focused on the gasps that never diminished, and I pulled a heavy side chair as close as I could.

After all the appointments (sometimes one every day), office visits, surgical procedures, medication schedules, late-night phone calls, ministrokes, bandages, scares, ambulance rides, and advocating—after all the effort that had gone into helping one cherished human being leave this world in peace—my mom was lying next to me, gasping for air with sounds I'll never forget. Meanwhile, a nurse lingered outside the room, incapable of granting a gentle passage.

Then there was no noise—just silence. The shock of silence was almost as startling as the loud breathing that had preceded it. I remembered what the hospice nurse had told me earlier in the day, and I knew my mother would start breathing—*I had to continue breathing.* But my mother never breathed again. She was forever silent. I kissed her cheek, and her skin was cool. At 11:00 P.M., I called my son.

* * *

My mom's confrontation with death occurred in an unfriendly, uncompromising setting with little assistance or comfort extended to either of us—except from my dog at the foot of the bed. Writing of her mother's passing, memoirist Liz Schreier said, ". . . she was able to take control of some measure of her life, even if only the place and comfort of its ending. Surely, we all deserve that."[72]

In our search for meaning in life and mortality, we often imagine final acts of merciful compassion. Never could I have anticipated that, when my mother's time arrived, hospice professionals at her final assisted living facility would not be in attendance—or even alerted. Nothing in the literature or notes suggested that we might be left alone without a hospice nurse or staff member to comfort us during my mother's hours of struggle from life to death, and my passage from adult child to orphan.

A contributor to the "Modern Love" column of *The New York Times* wrote about her brother's admission to hospice and the medication doses dispensed as death neared: "morphine for pain, Haldol for nausea and Lorazepam for anxiety. Each floated in a medicine-dropper-topped bottle so that liquid relief could be applied to the patient's cheek."[73] My mother received no drops of merciful liquid from her caregivers—no relief except the cessation of her own breathing.

* * *

---

72. Liz Schreier, *Never Simple* (New York: Henry Holt, 2022), p. 246.
73. Michelle Friedman, "Time Out for One Last Act of Intimate Kindness," *New York Times,* August 21, 2022.

I removed the thin plastic oxygen tubing from my mom's nose. After a few minutes, I walked to the corridor, intending to notify the nurse that the death had occurred. I saw she was mixing up a dose of something. She told me she'd retrieved a single morphine pill from the facility's contingency supply and was preparing it to assist my mother. I did not yell, advocate, or cry—I simply remembered to *breathe.*

When I returned to my mom's room, the nurse entered and said she'd called hospice, and they'd arrive in an hour. We had to wait for a hospice nurse to declare that my mom, my cold mom, was dead. And the hospice nurse would call the funeral home.

My mother was at peace. I looked at her and asked what she wanted me to do. I didn't have to wonder. She'd want me to clean up the room. I began by tossing used tissues and the collection of half-empty Revlon Cherries in the Snow nail polish bottles into a wastebasket near the low bed. Then I slowly tried to organize clothes and the remaining personal items.

When the nurse came back, she walked to my mom's side, looked down, and saw the nail polish. She asked me if she could have the bottles. I was beyond caring about either the nurse or red polish. I said, "Yes."

● ● ●

Because the hospice night nurse didn't arrive until 1:30 A.M., my mother's death certificate reads "April 12, 2018"—nine days before her one hundredth birthday. Realizing she remembered my mother from a different facility, over a year before, the nurse searched through her omnipresent hospice laptop to read notes she'd written about the sharp-witted, sweet Lillian and her sense of humor.

The hospice nurse and I waited for the funeral home representative. After they'd prepared my mother's body, my dog and

I followed the gurney along the corridor, out the front door, and into the circular driveway—until it was placed in the hearse and disappeared into the misty night. My mama took her final ride.

When we returned to gather our belongings, we startled the facility's night nurse, who was rifling through the wastebasket in the bathroom. The next morning, I called the state's long-term care ombudsman to cancel the meeting with the assisted living facility's director, a meeting that was no longer warranted. She said she'd handle the issue of the nurse. I no longer responded.

• • •

I lost my mother moments before 11:00 P.M. on April 11, 2018. The hospice notes for April 12 read:

1:00 drive start
1:28 drive end
2:00 Time of death
3:30 Visit end

A comment about the "daughter" reported that I was grieving appropriately. As one of my virtual siblings in a private Facebook group posted, "I experienced a profound rush of relief that no new bad thing would ever happen . . ."[74]

• • •

Atul Gawande famously wrote:

All we ask is to be allowed to remain the writers of our own story. That story is ever changing. Over the course of our lives, we may encounter unimaginable difficulties. Our concern and desires may

---

74. Private Facebook page, April 29, 2022.

shift. But whatever happens, we want to retain the freedom to shape our own lives in ways consistent with our character and loyalties.[75]

My mother shaped the last chapter of her life by moving fifteen hundred miles north to be with her daughter. She entrusted her last years to me.

Eric Boice, whose mother, Joan, died five months after moving to an assisted living facility in Auburn, California, reports that after her death, his mother visited him frequently in his dreams. In those dreams, she was healthy and lucid and able to communicate. They talked. And Eric told her he was sorry "for not being the voice she needed, for not demanding more of the people that we trusted with her care."[76]

When we buried my mother's remains in Florida, I looked at my father's headstone and said, "I did the best I could," but in my heart, I knew that the eldercare grid had failed us. I might have been loud (as the owner of a small, freestanding assisted living facility had alleged), but I might not have been loud enough.

• • •

Two days after the death of Britain's Queen Elizabeth II, in September 2022, Patti Davis recalled private moments from 2004, following public memorial ceremonies for her father, President Ronald Reagan:

Driving home through dark quiet streets, I knew the river of grief that was waiting for me, and I knew I would have to cross it alone.

---

75. Atul Gawande, *Being Mortal: Medicine and What Matters in the End* (New York: Henry Holt, 2014), p. 140.

76. A. C. Thompson and Jonathan Jones, "Life and Death in Assisted Living," *Frontline*, aired July 29, 2013, on PBS.

My hope is that people remember . . . In the end, though they [the royal family] breathe rarefied air, they grapple as we all do with life and death, with the mystery of what it means to be human. When darkness falls, and they are alone, they sink into the same waters that everyone does when a loved one dies. And they wonder if they'll make it to the other side.[77]

• • •

Studying deaths from COVID-19, and grief surrounding deaths during the pandemic, Camilla Wortman, professor emerita at Stony Brook University, says, "We traditionally think about people having a good death where they are in a setting where they are free of pain, their loved ones are surrounding them and their loved ones can tell them how much they meant to them."[78] My mother was a resident of an otherwise highly regarded assisted living facility, enrolled in hospice, and not a victim of the pandemic, but she did not have a pain-free death.

Researchers have recently embraced the notion that those who grieve suboptimal deaths are at risk for prolonged grief disorder—lasting for a year or more.[79] Eight months after my mother died, my PCP was noticeably concerned when I told her I still cried every day. Implying that my grief was excessive, she handed me a prescription for an antidepressant, a referral to a team of therapists, and an appointment for a return clinic visit six weeks later. I kept the appointment but didn't fill the prescription.

I sorted pictures, planned a family graveside memorial in Florida, and found my own therapist. I changed doctors. Discussing

---

77. Patti Davis, "The Royal Grief the Public Will Not See," *New York Times*, September 10, 2022.

78. "Covid Deaths Left Big Holes in the Hearts of Loved Ones. All That Grief is Taking a Toll," *New York Times*, May 21, 2022.

79. Ibid.

excessive grief disorder, one pediatrician/journalist wrote, "Grief is personal, individual, idiosyncratic—but it is also public and universal."[80] When I recall the undesirable alternatives we faced, the unreasonably difficult path we followed, and the chronic weaknesses I observed in our country's assisted living and hospice systems, I still cry.

80. Perri Class, M.D., "We Will All Mourn, and We Will All Be Mourned," *New York Times,* June 6, 2022.

Afterword

Soon after my mother moved north in the spring of 2006, she began attending a series of weekly *Lechayim* (the Hebrew for "to life") lunches sponsored by Jewish Social Services. Before long, she was encouraging other residents of her independent living community to attend, and she gathered them together in time for their Monday-morning shuttle bus.

Always fashionable, my mom selected her outfit for what she called her "Monday meeting" on Sunday afternoon—a skirt or pants, matching jacket, and a hair bow or colorful hat. If I was in her apartment on Sunday, I'd have to approve her wardrobe selections.

The people at her usual corner of the *Lechayim* room became close friends, and my mother loved chatting with the married couple at the adjoining table. She called them "the doctor and his wife."

My mother flourished at spirited lunches—kosher menus, a new circle of friends, and enlightening programs (lectures, short films, or entertainment). I joined her as frequently as possible, and, while I was there, I helped serve the meals. When music was on the program—especially the group of "old-timers" who played swing music—my mom and I danced. Always the entertainer, she smiled and waved to her audience as we both tried to lead.

When my mother moved to her sixth and final assisted living facility, I recognized a name on one of the resident's doors. The wife of the doctor from the *Lechayim* lunches was also living there! During the long month of my mom's residence, I never saw the woman at any meal or activity. Sometimes, I spotted a private caregiver quietly sitting outside the room, and I assumed the sweet, friendly woman we'd known was confined to bed.

· · ·

In the hour before my mother died, the only person from the assisted living facility staff who talked to me was the nurse who eventually prepared a too-late dose of morphine and then asked me for my mother's bottles of nail polish. I remember that while I was waiting for the hospice nurse, I heard a beverage cart rattling through the hall, and I walked out of the room to ask for a drink of water.

Later, I left my mom's room to find trash bags—planning to sort items to toss or donate. I walked to the end of the hallway, where a small circle of off-duty staff stood chatting. One was the nurse who'd called me at 9:30 P.M. to say my mother wouldn't make it through the night. Because of the phone call, I knew his shift was over. He was the only assisted living staff person who said, "I'm sorry." That was all. Two words. No hug or an offer of a hug. I asked the group where I could find large plastic bags, and someone led me to a supply closet.

Much later, as I returned along the corridor, having just watched my mother's gurney leave the front of the building, I realized that someone had been sitting in a chair outside the room of the doctor's wife all evening. She looked up as I passed—looked directly at me—and said, "I'm very sorry." I said, "Thank you." She could not have known that the two women—my mom and her patient—had, only a few years before, dressed up, laughed, and hugged as they greeted each other and shared weekly *Lechayim* lunches.

* * *

I remembered something the state long-term care ombudsman had mentioned: Recent relicensing of the facility from a nursing home to an assisted living facility meant that locks would be installed on the residents' doors. Because I didn't want anyone to have access to our belongings, I approached the night nurse to ask for a key to my mother's room. Visibly surprised that I knew to ask, she located a key in her desk drawer. I watched as she locked the door and kept the key. I had no more reactions to give. I left.

The next morning, a friend met me to start gathering clothing and other personal items. As we approached the assisted living wing, we met the hospice social worker and the hospice nurse who'd visited my mom in the weeks before her death. The social worker had a small collection of rocks and handed me one.

I still keep the rock near my front door—a shiny gray stone, like the ones on the beach behind the house on the Atlantic where I spent my childhood. Smaller than my palm, the rock has a white tree etched onto one side, with one leaf falling toward the ground—a hospice logo, I think. The other side says *Remember*— and I do.

The social worker also handed me a card referring me to the hospice's "free grief services." A couple of days later, I called the telephone number on the card to speak with a hospice counselor. The phone was disconnected.

* * *

At home, I sorted through my mother's pictures and tried to assemble collages of photographs for my children and grandchildren.

Then I rearranged them and started all over. The pictures covered my dining room table the day a counselor from hospice arrived at my front door. (In fact, the photos remained in the same spot for over a year.)

I have no idea what I said to the hospice visitor. He never sat down or engaged me in a meaningful conversation, but I know I pointed out the assortment of my mom's images. I continue to suspect he was sent because someone knew I was starting to ask questions about the omission of help and guidance at the time of my mother's death.

On the first of May, a bill arrived from the ambulance service that had conveyed my mother from the hospital to her sixth and final assisted living bed on a cold March morning. Medicare wouldn't cover the charges because my mother was not officially reinstated at hospice until she was removed from the ambulance and physically present at the care facility. I mailed a check to the private ambulance company.

Four days later, I received a statement from a pharmacy at a CCRC my mother never entered—for a single morphine pill that was never dispensed. Apparently, the facility where she died replenished its contingency supply from a collaborating entity that was three miles east. I called to question the charges and did not pay the bill.

. . .

Somehow, I found the strength to file complaints with the state, against both hospice and the assisted living home, for (1) failure to carry out a plan of care, and (2) disregard of policy. The two complaints outlined the same series of events, and the wording was similar in both letters:

1. [The facility] and [the hospice organization] failed to carry out a plan of care:

The signed admission document for [the facility] states "Provide education to patient and caregivers to contact [hospice] before using comfort pack medications . . . Educate on comfort pack use. Identify comfort plan starting 3/12/2018."
Further Goals: "Patient will have plan for emergency medication needs through end of life."

But no morphine (no *comfort pack*) was available to ease my mother's final discomfort. This is a confusing situation: [Hospice] staff report that the end-of-life comfort pack always includes 10 morphine sulfate tablets (20 doses).

- There are handwritten notes on [hospice] records, in reference to three medications: lorazepam, hyoscyamine, and morphine: "Pharmacy: Please fill only after requested by facility."

- The [hospital geriatric clinic] reports that the note on the morphine was added because 30 pills (60 doses) of morphine had been ordered and delivered on March 16, 2018, but:

- [The packaging pharmacy] and control personnel report that morphine was *never* requested and never filled. (Apparently, the prescriptions for lorazepam and hyoscyamine had been filled and delivered, since lorazepam had been administered regularly, and I believe I watched both lorazepam and hyoscyamine administered to my mother on the night of her death.)

- On April 13, 2017, a day after my mother died, a single capsule of morphine sulfate was ordered from [another pharmacy] (not her pharmacy), and I subsequently received an invoice . . .

- In addition, there was confusion surrounding the timing of lorazepam doses. The [hospital geriatric clinic] reports an order was written for lorazepam every three hours on March 12, 2018.

- Standing Orders for [the assisted living facility], signed March 16, 2018: "Suction as needed to clear airway." None was available. My mother received no help in clearing her airway, except for a probing via a sponge swab, which I observed about an hour before her death.

2. [Hospice] policies were disregarded:

- "Educate on comfort pack use."
- "Support patient/family in discussing and sharing feelings/ concerns related to approaching death."
- "Family demonstrates their understanding of what to expect during the dying process and what to do at time of death."
  - I did not know that there was no morphine available for my mother in her last struggle.
  - I did not know there was no suction bulb syringe available. At 10:15 at night, I offered to drive to an all-night pharmacy to purchase one.
- [Hospice] team personnel never engaged me in a discussion about the end-of-life process. They did not know that I had never witnessed a transition to death. (I initiated a discussion about characteristic breathing with the itinerant [hospice] nurse, in the hours preceding my mother's death, out of curiosity about comments I had solicited from a grieving friend.)

I received two letters from the state. The first, regarding the assisted living facility, read, in part:

Surveyors conducted an onsite complaint investigation . . . A tour of the provider location or facility; observation of care; a review of records; interview with residents and families; and interviews with provider/facility staff.

As a result of the investigation there was not enough evidence to confirm that a violation of the regulations occurred related to your concerns. Our investigation does not in any way discount your observations or experiences. It means only that we were unable to prove that this provider violated state and or federal regulations related to your concerns.

The second letter (referring to hospice) read, in part:

A surveyor . . . conducted an onsite investigation that concluded on July 25, 2018. The investigation included a review of medical records, policies, the complaint file, staff interviews, and observations.

As a result of our investigation, we confirmed the factual basis for your concerns. However, the facts and circumstances do not constitute a violation of Wisconsin Statutes or Administrative Code (and/ or Medicare requirements). Therefore, this office issued no statement of deficiency against the facility relative to your complaint.

• • •

I submitted the facts as I had experienced the events, and the state had the last word—almost. When I met with the funeral home personnel, they asked me the usual difficult questions about death certificates and how many copies I thought I'd need. I had no idea, so I ordered too many.

When the documents arrived, I read through the words that told me my mother was legally gone. Due to the delayed call to hospice and the after-midnight appearance of a hospice nurse, the "pronounced dead" date reads "April 12, 2018," not April 11, 2018, the date on which I watched and heard my mother die.

The immediate cause was listed as "ASPIRATION PNEUMO-NIA." Indeed, that had been the cause of her final months of struggle. The other significant condition was listed as "ALZHEIM-ER'S DISEASE."

I stared at the official wording for several days and finally called my mother's PCP, who'd, apparently, made the cause-of-death determination. "Please, help," I said. "For the last fifteen months, I attempted to maintain hospice coverage and was told that my mother wasn't dying fast enough—because she *wasn't* suffering from Alzheimer's." If my mother hadn't been dying from what they said she wasn't dying from, how could she have ultimately died because of it?

The death certificates were reprinted, and I received new copies from the county registrar of deeds. The "other significant condition" was recorded as "VASCULAR DEMENTIA." My mother and I contributed the last words.

The system tried to contain her, and, until the end, my mother remained aware of the failings. She held her own as long as she could—until she was just nine days away from turning one hundred.

. . .

The afternoon after my mother's death, the rabbi from Jewish Social Services guided me through my visit to the funeral home. When we met at a neighborhood coffee shop a few weeks later, we talked about a family memorial service in Florida, next to my father's grave site. The rabbi suggested we read a poem.

Because I was still consoling myself by selecting images to share with my children, I walked back from the coffee shop and continued sifting through an old brown envelope that was filled with sepia-tone family pictures. I found a fragile page from a school notebook tucked in the bottom of the envelope. Faded handwritten phrases had been inscribed there by my mother's younger sister, who'd died while still in high school.

When we gathered on July 1, 2018, one day after my seventy-sixth birthday, my family and two lifelong friends read a poem written by the aunt I never knew:

> Oh to be alone some lonely night
> When the moon shines on the world so bright
> While the breeze blows softly through your hair

Relieving your mind of all despair
As soft dew grass circles your feet
And a maple stump serves as your seat
While you listen much to your dismay
To a woodland concert about to play
Then, as if a maestro's magic wand
Releases its prey from a silent bond
Music quickly fills the tranquil night
As birds and beetles their songs unite[81]

* * *

Faced with stark truths about the frailty of our long-term care industry and its inability to protect our most precious and vulnerable population—notably during a public health crisis, as we would see during the COVID-19 pandemic—we must activate to promote change. For eldercare, for the physical and emotional health and dignity of all, we have to rethink our patronage of the high-growth, high-margin real estate business known as assisted living, as well as the federal government benefit that provides hospice service to a population expected to die within six months.

We cannot continue relying on a deficient and undervalued staffing model, and we must recognize and legitimize family angst and advocacy.

---

81. Written by Frances Cowan, age sixteen or seventeen (circa 1938 or 1939).

Conclusion

This book records our personal story. Within the background of recent financial history, my mother and I represented a microcosm. Our journey mirrored trends in long-term care and the broader housing market for the early decades of the twenty-first century.

Because I'd recently participated in a study of investment in seniors housing, I thought I knew all that was relevant about the long-term care economic model. But my understanding was limited to investment feasibility, while the real world is broader than basic dollars and cents. In time, the stage became populated with authentic lives, including ours.

• • •

In the spring of 2007, more than six years before I became a daily visitor to assisted living facilities, Elaine Worzala, a friend and colleague, who was then serving as professor of real estate in the Edward St. John Real Estate Program at Johns Hopkins University, contacted me about joining her and Jeffrey Davis, founder and CEO of Cambridge Realty Capital Companies, to assist in researching, writing, and editing a white paper on institutional investing in seniors housing.

All three of us had received graduate degrees from the real estate program at the University of Wisconsin–Madison School of Business, and we'd been drilled in finance and feasibility analysis by the revered Professor James Graaskamp. Elaine and Jeff had already submitted a funding proposal to the Real Estate Research Institute (RERI), illuminating the project's objectives:

> The elderly housing sector has expanded in response to changing demographics and the increased needs of an ageing population. As the baby boomers reach retirement age and move into their "sunshine" years, the demand for real estate product that is designed with this elderly end user in mind is growing and risk/return profiles of these investments are shifting. Despite the incredible and expected growth, there has been little focused research on this alternative asset class from the perspective of an institutional investor. Research results will assist the investment community as they begin to invest in this unique real estate investment.[82]

Looking back, I realize how unaware I was of key physical and financial characteristics of assisted living facilities—either as a student of real estate investment or an adult child/potential consumer.

* * *

Before we began our work, Jeff insisted that Elaine and I visit eight or ten long-term care facilities in our respective areas. Every organization, from the Alzheimer's Association and the American Association of Retired Persons (AARP) to the state of Wisconsin's

---

82. Elaine Worzala, Judith F. Karofsky, and Jeffrey A. Davis, "An Exploration of the Risk and Return Spectrum for Institutional Investors," Proposal Abstract (2007).

Aging and Disability Resource Centers (ADRC) and Department of Health Services (DHS), recommends visiting several facilities before formulating life-changing decisions. They all publish lists of suggestions entitled "What to ask" or "What to look for."

Families tend to make choices based on proximity and whether neighbors, relatives, or friends are already residents. Indeed, when my mother moved north, we visited four well-known residences and selected one within walking distance of my home—where I was familiar with current and former occupants and their families. However, as my life moved forward, Jeff's assignment proved increasingly valuable.

By 2009, when our white paper was published in the *Journal of Real Estate Portfolio Management,* the seemingly endless housing expansion of 2002 to 2006 had begun to reverse. Economists and pundits who observed and commented on the economy and its effects on older people reported that seniors were realizing lower proceeds from home sales, and some were unwilling to sell at all. Aging baby boomers were seeking more affordable options—remaining where they were or downsizing—and they were delaying or cutting back on spending for congregate housing. Investment risk for long-term care properties was perceived as trending upward.

When published, both the "Executive Summary" and "Conclusion" of the white paper reflected the sea change in the economy. Instead of proposing to "assist the investment community as they begin to invest in [a] unique real estate investment," the study morphed into overt encouragement for investment in an undervalued but essential real estate sector:

> *We queried members of the Pension Real Estate Association to determine how they view this property sector compared with alternative real estate investments, as well as more traditional institutional investments, such as stocks and bonds. We found that*

they do not appear to be investing in most of the seniors housing product available, as they perceive it to have relatively high risk, and they do not perceive the returns to be high compared to more traditional real estate investments or alternative investments like international real estate.[83]

We reported the results of a survey of plan sponsor members of the Pension Real Estate Association. Respondents had been asked their opinions about "risk and return levels associated with the seniors housing sectors in comparison to more traditional real estate investments and to more conventional financial assets, including stocks and bonds."[84]

The results of the survey show clearly that members of the pension fund investment community are not currently invested nor are they looking to invest in seniors housing. They rate the risks higher than some of the other more traditional real estate investments but the returns lower than some of the alternative investments that might be considered relatively risky, such as international real estate investments. We believe this mismatch of risk and return levels is due to a lack of understanding of the seniors housing subsectors and hope this research provides a picture of the market and will allow for a better understanding of the seniors housing investment alternatives. . . . As more investors consider seniors housing, they will give this property type a higher degree of scrutiny and hopefully expand investments, given the ever-increasing need for new development as our population continues to age.[85]

---

83. Elaine Worzala, Judith F. Karofsky, Jeffrey A. Davis. "The Senior Living Property Sector: How Is It Perceived by the Institutional Investor?" *Journal of Real Estate Portfolio Management* 15, no. 2 (2009):141.

84. Ibid., p. 155.

85. Ibid., p.154.

One reviewer of the white paper wrote:

> Investments in seniors housing may not be as risky as earlier per-
> ceived, according to a newly released study, which also shows
> financial returns in this specialized real estate sector on a par with
> more traditional property types. . . . the study could spark an atti-
> tude change among institutional investors and generate new capi-
> tal for the seniors housing industry.[86]

● ● ●

Our work had ongoing relevance. For several years, Jeff Davis remained interested in researching and reporting how perceptions of risk and reward in the seniors housing business models were evolving with improvements in the overall housing economy. Unfortunately, by then, my view became inner-directed: I was enmeshed in the real-time saga of my mom's progression through assisted living and long-term care. Crisis by crisis, I began to tally our needs, the personal risks of her failing health, and the personal costs of our constant stress.

On one hand, I was a trained observer of perceived risk and reward as they affect financial decision making in an essential industry; on the other, I was a daughter and advocate for an aging parent in assisted living facilities. While demographic projections called for increased supply, and our research indicated that insti-tutional investments could be encouraged by calculating and pub-lishing ongoing risk-return data, my real-life experiences produced a cynical view of the existing long-term care industry. Personal observations and instincts led me to question whether familiar seniors housing real estate models worked any longer.

---

86. Jane Adler, "New Study Debunks Myths about Investment Risks in Seniors Housing," *National Real Estate Investor,* May 28, 2008. https:// www.nreionline.com/seniors-housing/new-study-debunks-myths -about-investment-risks-seniors-housing

. . .

Although assisted living offers housing, food, activities, and limited hours of professional care for aging residents who do not require skilled nursing—as well as respite for families and relatives—the facilities remain commercial enterprises that must remain solvent to survive.

Whether I was meeting with owners and managers, spending long days within the walls of assisted living facilities and memory care units, or sharing the confusion and pain of other adult children, I remained aware of the underlying business model: the ongoing needs to raise capital, cover costs, mitigate financial threats, enhance the bottom line, and maximize dollars per square foot.

. . .

In 2009, the publication year of our work, the housing economy fell victim to the Great Recession that followed the financial crisis of 2007–2008 and the U.S. subprime mortgage crisis of 2007–2009. Investment resources were limited, and bank assets were collapsing—or threatening to collapse—until the financial sector was bailed out by the U.S. government.

Within the seniors housing universe, the specific question was whether risks due to care, management, and service provision were too great to incentivize needed investments in assisted living and memory care—compared to the projected rewards of more familiar investments in independent living and age restricted (over-fifty-five) apartments.

. . .

As a microdata point, when my mother began her stay in independent living in the spring of 2006, only three of the six assisted living facilities where she'd eventually reside even existed. (As if anticipating my mom's forthcoming moves among assisted living facilities, the other three opened between 2013 and 2017.)

In 2008, as my coauthors and I engaged in our research, beds in Wisconsin nursing homes still outnumbered those in assisted living facilities. Over the next decade, as the demographic wave started to churn, skilled nursing homes became mired in increased costs and regulations—and less reliable Medicaid reimbursements—and assisted living broke through as a more attractive investment. As one officer of an association representing both nursing homes and assisted living facilities said, "It's incredibly expensive to run a nursing facility these days."[87]

By the time my mother moved to her sixth assisted living facility, in March 2018—precisely when the license category was in the process of being changed from skilled nursing to assisted living—there was a proliferation of over one hundred assisted living options in the county, and many more in the development pipeline. Countywide, only eighteen skilled nursing facilities remained, and additional closures or conversions to assisted living were being discussed.

Investment capital had found its way to assisted living—the segment of the long-term care sector that offers attractive, marketable activities; where financial risk (perceived as onerous in skilled nursing homes) is mitigated by the absence of federal oversight and relatively few state regulations; and where labor cost containment can be achieved by hiring CNAs, instead of licensed nurses, in many areas.

● ● ●

---

87. David Wahlberg, "Converting Nursing Home to Assisted Living, a Possible Trend," *The Wisconsin State Journal*, October 30, 2017.

In April 2018, as my mother lay dying in a Wisconsin assisted living facility, a coalition of health care organizations reported that the state's shortage of long-term care personnel continued to deepen—even after the Wisconsin Assisted Living Association (WALA) had issued a warning two years before:

> A caregiver vacancy report issued in 2016 confirmed the existence of a workforce crisis confronting long-term and residential care providers. This report, based on data from a 2018 survey of 756 providers, reveals a continuing crisis due in part to:
> - Fewer caregivers entering the workforce
> - Increasing number of people seeking long-term care and residential care
> - Continued growth in demand for caregivers
> - Gaps in the starting wage for entry level personal caregivers and non-healthcare workers
> - Wisconsin's Medicaid reimbursement system does not cover the cost of care incurred by long-term care providers
> - Wisconsin's historically low unemployment rate
>
> The results of this survey substantiate the continued workforce crisis facing providers who serve persons needing long-term and residential care and reinforce the need for public/private efforts to overcome this significant challenge.[88]

Attributing the crisis to caregivers leaving jobs for higher pay elsewhere and retirements of licensed practical nurses (LPNs) and registered nurses (RNs), the study reported that one-fifth of

---

88. Wisconsin Health Care Association/Wisconsin Center for Assisted Living, Wisconsin Assisted Living Association, LeadingAge Wisconsin, Disability Service Provider Network, "The Long-Term Care Workforce Crisis: A 2018 Report," https://www.leadingagewi.org/media/53421/workforce-report-2018.pdf.

providers were experiencing staff vacancy rates of at least 30 percent. "84% of the time providers rely on overtime, double shifts, and other financial strategies to fill open hours—expensive options that can lead to caregiver burnout."[89]

• • •

For four and a half years, I experienced an adult child's worst nightmares when I waited for help, performed difficult tasks—like transferring my exhausted mother into bed—or wandered anxiously through empty assisted living facility hallways, looking for caregivers.

The WALA study failed to mention increased demand for staff that was generated by introducing new assisted living facilities into the market. I was no longer officially reviewing data from the National Investment Center for Seniors Housing & Care (NIC) on "analytics and insights that investors and operators need to make informed decisions,"[90] but I listened to staff members as they discussed and responded to news that yet another assisted living facility was being added to the inventory. Although pay was low and benefits were rare, open solicitation encouraged employee migration. Caregivers, nurses, and senior staff were attracted to every assisted living facility's grand opening.

• • •

Not quite two years after my mother's death, a worldwide pandemic forced assisted living facilities to expand their role beyond

---

89. Wisconsin Health Care Association/Wisconsin Center for Assisted Living, Wisconsin Assisted Living Association, LeadingAge Wisconsin, Disability Service Provider Network, "The Long-Term Care Workforce Crisis: A 2018 Report," https://www.leadingagewi.org/media/53421 /workforce-report-2018.pdf.

90. https://www.nic.org.

conventional safety precautions, minimal health care, and social activities:

> As the full scope of the COVID-19 threat became apparent in early 2020, federal, state, and local policymakers acted to mitigate the spread of the virus in the community and within congregate living settings. Although federal and state governments jointly regulate nursing care provided in skilled nursing facilities, assisted living is state-regulated and independent living is, in most states, not regulated. As a result, operators faced myriad restrictions from senior housing care segment, property to property, state to state, and county to county.[91]

The virus was more devastating for the elderly than for their children.

> In the first half of 2020, as understanding grew about the scope of COVID-19's impact on seniors housing, many properties instituted infection control policies to protect residents and reduce the spread of the virus. Such policies included restricting visitors, halting communal dining and group activities, cohorting residents and staff, and reinventing physical spaces and workflow processes to include safely donning and doffing PPE.[92]

The seniors housing industry is bottom line–oriented (exactly what we'd been trying to articulate when we focused our 2008–2009 study on risk, reward, and investment decision making) and the industry was caught unprepared.

---

91. NORC at the University of Chicago and National Investment Center for Seniors Housing and Care (NIC), *The Impact of COVID-19 on Seniors Housing, Final Report,* June 3, 2021, p. 10, https://www.norc.org/research/projects/the-impact-of-covid-19-on-senior-housing.html
92. Ibid., p. 3.

In 1981, UW-Madison Professor Jim Graaskamp wrote:

> Foreseeable future trends have many subtle impacts on real estate development. . . . . As these added costs modify the pricing structure and trade-off issues for the real estate consumer, the defined competitive standard will begin to shift. . . . Notice that the ability to internalize these requirements in the capital cost/monthly payments and therefore the cash cycle of the user begins to provide an infinite number of trade-off decisions for the developer, the consumer, and the public agencies regulating the development process.[93]

But the pandemic's impact was *not* subtle. On September 20, 2020, *The New York Times* editorial board wrote:

> Around 40 percent of all coronavirus-related deaths in the United States have been among the staff and residents of nursing homes and other long-term care facilities—totaling some 68,000 people.
>
> Some 70 percent of America's long-term care facilities are run by for-profit companies, including private investment firms. Those companies have squeezed profits out of these facilities by forcing them to skimp on care.[94]

Suddenly, financial data was illustrated with personal pain. By March 31, 2021, the COVID Tracking Project reported:

> Residents of nursing homes and other long-term care facilities suffered an outsized impact from COVID-19. What we . . . know makes it plain that we failed to protect this community—and at great cost.

---

93. James A. Graaskamp, *Fundamentals of Real Estate Development* (Washington, D.C.: Urban Land Institute, 1981), p.29

94. "A Damning New York Times Editorial Slams Nursing Home Industry," *SEIU Healthcare*, September 15, 2020.

Despite making up less than 1% of the nation's population, people living in nursing homes and other long-term care (LTC) facilities account for *at least* 35% of the nation's COVID-19 deaths.[95]

1. We did not protect the vulnerable

. . . The residents of long-term care facilities were by far the most vulnerable of all US populations throughout the pandemic's first year—and they were not by any measure protected until vaccines finally began to reach them in late December, nearly 10 months after the first known outbreak of COVID-19 in a US long-term care facility.

2. Our failure to protect LTC [Long Term Care] residents resulted in staggering losses

. . . as of March 2021, about 8 percent of people who live in US long-term care facilities have died of COVID-19: Nearly one in 12. For nursing homes alone, the figure is nearly one in 10.

3. We still don't know the full toll of the pandemic on LTC residents and workers

. . . Federal data on COVID-19 in nursing homes covers only skilled nursing facilities, and excludes the experience of approximately 800,000 people living in assisted living facilities and similar residential care communities. . . . we believe that the true toll of the pandemic among these workers and especially residents is higher than these figures can show.[96]

• • •

---

95. The COVID Tracking Project, https://covidtracking.com/analysis -updates/what-we-know-about-the-impact-of-the-pandemic-on-our -most-vulnerable-community.

96. Ibid.

Going forward, investment in the long-term care industry will have to address previously unforeseen problems and estimate the economic fallout of ever greater risks.

The pandemic necessitated fundamental shifts in processes, workflow, and operational thinking to keep residents and staff safe. As stay-at-home orders were issued, operators had to adapt to keep their properties appropriately staffed to meet the social and medical needs of residents. Many operators took an "all hands on deck" approach to staffing—for example, transportation personnel became temperature checkers and physical therapists became resident window visitors. . . . Operators also restricted visitation and halted communal dining and other group activities. Social activities, such as music and games that were previously held in group settings were adapted to limit contact. Building layouts, described by many operators as communal and social in nature, required swift adaptation to implement infection control protocols as the pandemic unfolded. Operators created COVID-19 isolation rooms, COVID-19 positive "communities," and move-in quarantine wings, as well as staff cohorts to focus on different segments of the property to mitigate the close contact interactions between staff and residents.[97]

● ● ●

Although "occupied units plummeted until January 2021 and then began to recover with the introduction of the vaccine,"[98]

---

97. NORC at the University of Chicago and National Investment Center for Seniors Housing and Care (NIC), *The Impact of COVID-19 on Seniors Housing, Final Report,* June 3, 2021, p. 18, https://www.norc.org/research/projects/the-impact-of-covid-19-on-senior-housing.html

98. Daniel G. Lindberg, "The Price Elasticity of Senior Housing Demand: Is It a Necessity or a Luxury?" National Association for Business Economics, October 21, 2022, https://pmc.ncbi.nlm.nih.gov/articles/PMC9589560/

long-term care industry publications continued to announce purchases and sales of portfolios of assisted living facilities. As before, relevant metrics were based on price per living unit—sometimes, price per bed. Investors respond to demographic forecasts and projected demand, and in the inflationary economy, purchase prices of assisted living facilities continued to rise.

Management and operations are key to assisted living facilities' economic performance. Speaking broadly of health care innovations in 2022, Dr. Nicholas Holmes, COO, Rady Children's Hospital, San Diego, said, "When the pandemic came along, it really changed the lens of how we do health care design . . . And what we learned over the past few years, first and foremost, is to be as flexible . . . as possible."[99]

For 2022,

> The lower occupancy for majority assisted living facilities [compared to a majority of units in independent living] saw rates [rents] decline while expenses—particularly labor—grew by nearly 6% despite fewer residents. . . . for majority assisted living, the confluence of lower occupancy, lower revenues per occupied unit and rapidly rising expenses led to a 26% decline in net operating income (NOI) per occupied unit and margin drop from 30% to 22%.[100]

• • •

The risks are ongoing. The physical environment, emotional atmosphere, and financial underpinnings of long-term care all have changed. The U.S. Department of Health and Human Services has created a series of social media graphics and videos aimed at congregate living: "In long-term care, your risk for severe flu,

---

99. Debra Kamin, "Redesigning Hospitals for Greater Flexibility," *New York Times*, September 14, 2002.

100. *The State of Seniors Housing 2022* (Washington, D.C.: American Seniors Housing Association), p. 15.

COVID-19, or RSV is higher—vaccines help keep serious illness out of your plans."[101]

Postpandemic health threats to a vulnerable population will have to be contained—at a cost. In the new market reality, owners and investors will need to anticipate, identify, and manage infectious diseases and the potentially devastating progression of life-threatening symptoms. They will have to pivot toward contactless innovations, redesigned common areas, four-season outdoor rooms, private eating spaces, increased bandwidth, improved air quality, and new employment models—and they will realize less predictable investment returns.

Consumers' prices for long-term care will rise, and prices for the consistent quality care that should have been provided all along will rise even more. This story line does not end well.

• • •

It is time to change the narrative. We need a national dialogue on assisted living facilities that will address everything from post-COVID-19 room configuration to caregiver supply, both state and federal oversight, affordability, and industry consolidation. The well-capitalized institutional community—funded through REITs, private equity, or public pension funds—can develop the real estate, institute operational improvements, and oversee marketing details that will increase the supply of this necessity across the nation, but the trade-off is that large-scale investments *diminish accountability.*[102]

---

101. hhs.gov/risk-less-do-more/campaign-ads/index.html.

102. In an ironic twist, ". . . robust [private equity] returns benefit public pension funds and their beneficiaries, including millions of schoolteachers, public servants, and first responders who rely on them to strengthen their retirements." American Investment Council, "Private Equity & Main Street: New Report Highlights Middle Market Investment," September 17, 2024.

The farther the corporate decision-makers are from our seniors housing communities and their inhabitants, the more unlikely we will be to achieve a consistent assisted living mission of *compassionate care for the elderly.*[103] Our parents and grandparents are not mere digits. Consumers (aging residents and their families) have complex problems and interconnected lives that are messy and might not be easily programmed. Our obligation is to work together to create and advance a care plan that will honor the defenseless and protect our most vulnerable.

---

103. Private equity has already made inroads into the nursing home industry—with tragic results and loss of life. In the book *Plunder: Private Equity's Plan to Pillage America,* and an article, "Private Equity Is Gutting America and Getting Away with It" (*New York Times*, April 30, 2023), Brendan Ballou argues: "By making equity firms responsible for their own actions, we can build a better—and fairer—economy and make tragedies . . . less likely. All we need is the courage to act."

Acknowledgments

It took a *New Village*:

This book is dedicated to my virtual siblings in courage—the members of a private Facebook group—over seven hundred graduates of Bryn Mawr College who are or have been struggling with unanticipated commonalities: age, family entanglements, terminal illnesses, dementia, hospice, and grief. I've been an administrator (a modern lantern person). Nothing here relates to late-night study sessions in Rhoads North, but let us share. *Anassa kata.*

This work happened because of the CNAs, nurses, chefs, physical therapists, physicians, hospice volunteers, receptionists, and activities staff who worked with and loved my mother. You know who you are, Jessica.

We traveled this far because my soul mate and bicycle guru, Andy M., repeatedly told me that book publication moves at glacial speed. My personal poet laureate, Jodi, similarly said, "The road to publishing is long, but important material finds its way."

I would have nothing to save without the tech support of Jason and Brenda H. And my home would not have remained my productive workspace without Brenda B. and Darrin.

I am forever grateful to Elaine W. and Jeff, who invited me to join a study of investment in seniors housing. Also, to our beloved "Chief", who taught us that real estate was created when the first individual rolled a rock in front of a cave—an historic precursor to the late-twentieth-century introduction of assisted living as a care concept where residents could shut their doors and lock their rooms.

My well-connected friends Melanie and Caryl were the first to confirm that the long-term care industry has widespread failings, and my former colleague Betsy reminded me not to write in anger. Mark C. and Lynn accompanied me until all my mother's personal items were accounted for.

These bouquets belong to Bonnie, Lana, and David S., who do not know one another, but who traveled almost parallel paths to mine, accompanying their beautiful mothers. And, of course, to Dave A., whose family needed and deserved more compassionate care.

My journey was accomplished safely because friends communicated by phone as I returned from my mom's assisted living facilities, driving over icy roads on dark nights: Eve, Nadine, and my daughter-in-law, Monica.

Many memories remain because of those who knew my mom longest and lived our story: my cousins, Gary, Andrew, and Joanne; my lifelong friends, Loretta, Stephen, and Mark G. (who was starkly honest after reading an early draft); and my childhood neighbor, Ron, who said, "Write for an hour every day." (And I did.)

This story was extended by my AC family, who allowed me to remain healthy during the pandemic and continue social distancing, even after vaccinations eased our fears—to write, send out queries, and miss my own birthday party: Craig, Mushka, Joe, David P., and two Nates.

This prayer is chanted with Rabbi Renee.

My emotional strength to stay on target was shared with Erri. My physical strength, with Septi.

These words were crafted with encouragement and understanding from Eve, enhanced by creative caffeinated hours with my writing partner Meredith, and prodded by sage coaching from the prolific mystery writer John. They had faith.

This song is sung for Francie and Mike, who led us *Over the Rainbow* on April 12, 2018, and to everyone else who was in the room hugging me—especially Josh, the birthday girl Robin, Shira, J.P., Rick, and Jay. And of course, Bridget, who insisted I walk to the Ivory on that holy night.

The task was accomplished with interest from my student neighbors who noticed me working in my bay window: Riley, Tess, Morgan, Maïa, and Carol—and from my gentle and beautiful pamperers: Olive, Jessica, Madeleine, Jennifer, and Aubrey.

An impromptu breakfast club (Steve, Rebecca, Heather, Nate M., Dan, and Jeff) kept my body and soul nourished through the final revisions. The wrap came with reassurance from my publisher Lynne and her wise staff and editors; a typically long lunch with Elaine D.; a title list from Harvey; a cover concept from Mushka; notes from Norm; legal eyes from two Jameses; kindness from my once and always governor; cheerleading from Kelly; webcrafting by JJ; publicity shots from Tim and Kevin; and final readings by Amy, Denise, and Elaine W. An unplanned meet-up with David H., who reminded me of the dangerous flaws we witnessed as concerned children, afforded my final resolve.

My heart is filled with Nana Lil's legacy of love: my three children, Jill, Amy, and Andy K.; my grandchildren: Daphne, Logan, Danny, Campbell, and McKerrah; my sons-in-law; and my daughter-in-law (my sounding board, assistant producer, and spell checker) and her parents, Lydia and Joseph—with unbounded thanks to Amy, my editor on call.

Glossary

Ageism
Prejudice towards older people. The act of stereotyping, demeaning, or discriminating against those who are no longer young.

Alzheimer's disease
A progressive, neurodegenerative disease characterized by memory loss, disorientation, mood swings, and the inability to care for oneself.

Administrative code
The compiled rules and regulations promulgated by a state's governmental agencies.

Aspiration pneumonia
A lung infection demonstrated by a persistent, debilitating cough. Occurs more often in elderly people who suffer from defective or impaired swallowing ability.

Assisted living
Housing for seniors that includes rooms, meals, limited health attention, and activities—for those who are still mobile and not in need of skilled nursing. Licensed and regulated by the individual states.

Caregiver stress
Adverse emotional and physical effects on the health and wellbeing of relatives and loved ones who oversee either in-home or institutional patient care.

Centers for Medicare & Medicaid Services (CMS)
The federal agency within the U.S. Department of Health and Human Services (HHS) that administers Medicare and works with individual states to administer Medicaid and the Health Insurance Portability and Accountability Act (HIPAA). Establishes and monitors quality standards for nursing homes but not for assisted living or memory care facilities.

Certified Nursing Assistant (CNA)
A healthcare worker who provides basic care, usually under the supervision of a licensed or registered nurse.

Comfort pack
The emergency kit supplied by a hospice organization to the caregivers of every patient. Contains small amounts of medicines available for common end-of-life symptoms, without necessitating additional prescriptions.

Community-based residential facility (CBRF)
Housing for seniors that offers nursing availability, housekeeping, meals, and progressive care as residents' needs increase. Licensed and regulated by the individual states.

Continuing care retirement community (CCRC)
A comprehensive complex that provides continuity of care for seniors. Starting with independent living, medical and accommodation options allow residents to remain on the same campus when their needs change. Licensed and regulated by the individual states.

COVID-19
An infectious coronavirus disease caused by the SARS-CoV-2 virus. The COVID-19 pandemic was declared by the World Health Organization (WHO) on March 11, 2020. This highly contagious acute respiratory disease was especially dangerous for older adults who were housed in congregate care.

Do not resuscitate (DNR)
A standing order indicating that a person should not receive cardiopulmonary resuscitation (CPR) if that person's heart stops beating.

Haloperidol (Haldol)
A behavior modification drug commonly used to treat nervous, emotional, and mental conditions. Not approved for older adults suffering from dementia.

Health Insurance Portability and Accountability Act (HIPAA)
The U.S. law prohibiting healthcare providers and businesses from disclosing protected information to anyone other than the patient and authorized representatives, without the patient's consent.

Hospice
A for-profit or nonprofit agency that offers a multidisciplinary team of professionals who provide palliative care, emotional support, essential supplies, and carefully selected medicines to the terminally ill—in homes, long-term care facilities, or hospitals. Funded and regulated by Medicare for patients expected to live six months or less.

Hospitalist
A doctor who only provides care for hospitalized patients.

Hoyer lift
A device designed to reduce the strain of repositioning patients with mobility challenges. Consists of a U-shaped base, an overhead bar, and a sling that lifts and lowers a patient to a chair, toilet, or bed.

Independent living
Congregate housing for seniors that offers rooms or apartments, activities, and meal plans. Residents manage their own health care and medications.

Kosher food
According to definitions rooted in the Bible, food fit for a Jewish person to eat.

Lorazepam (Ativan)
A drug used to reduce agitation and treat seizures and anxiety disorders.

Med passer
An unlicensed caregiver who meets state requirements to be able to administer medications to assisted living, memory care, and nursing home residents, as well as to hospice patients.

Medicaid
The U.S. government program that provides health insurance for adults and children with limited resources. Covers long-term costs for nursing

home and personal care services. Primarily managed and partially funded by the individual states.

Medicare
The U.S. health insurance program that provides health care for people aged 65 or older, plus younger people with certain disabilities. Covers hospital, skilled nursing, and rehabilitation services for limited periods of time. Reimburses hospice organizations for care and supplies. Does not pay for assisted living or memory care.

Memory care
A subset of assisted living that offers programming for those suffering from Alzheimer's disease or other dementias and provides security to prevent residents from wandering. Licensed and regulated by the individual states.

Morphine
An opioid prescribed in hospice care to manage discomfort at the end of life. Can reduce pain and ease breathing. Not intended to hasten death.

Obsessive-compulsive disorder (OCD)
A behavioral condition in which individuals attempt to relieve anxiety by constantly repeating phrases, acts, or routines.

Ombudsman
A government employee charged with investigating and attempting to resolve complaints or impasses that include public authorities. Involves recommendations, collaboration, and mediation.

Oxycodone (OxyContin)
An extended-release synthetic opioid used to treat moderate to severe pain. Highly addictive.

Physical therapy (PT)
A nonsurgical treatment protocol employing exercises and other techniques to reduce pain and correct a medical problem.

Pivot disc
A rotating disc that is placed on the floor to make transfers easier for users with limited mobility. Requires one helper or assistant.

Primary care physician (PCP)
The physician who cares for an individual's ongoing medical conditions. The first contact for undiagnosed health concerns.

Private equity
An investment approach that adopts an active role in the purchase, management, and re-structuring of target companies. Does not offer stock to the general public.

Real estate investment trust (REIT)
A financial entity that acquires and manages a diversified portfolio of income-producing real estate assets, offering significant dividends and tax advantages to investors. Usually trades on major stock exchanges.

Residential care apartment complex (RCAC)
Seniors housing that consists of independent apartments, each of which has a unique, lockable entrance and exit, and usually includes a meal plan. Licensed and regulated by the individual states.

Skilled nursing
Patient care that requires advanced training, such as post-operative care.

Skilled nursing facility (nursing home)
A facility providing either short-term or long-term skilled nursing care. Depending on circumstances, costs may be covered by Medicare or Medicaid. Licensed and monitored by the federal government.

Sundowning
The state of confusion, restlessness, and combativeness that occurs in late afternoon and lasts into evening for people suffering from Alzheimer's disease or dementia.

Transient ischemic attack (TIA)
A temporary stroke, or ministroke, presenting with weakness or numbness on one side of the body, vision loss, confusion, and/or limited speech. Frequently a precursor to a major stroke.

Vascular dementia
Dementia attributed to one or several small strokes, as dying brain cells result in permanent damage.

About the Author

Judy Karofsky was one of Wisconsin's first women mayors. During her term of office in the city of Middleton, she established a now-thriving senior center and emergency medical services. She served on the executive staff of a governor and held multiple roles in housing and economic development for a state agency, a nonprofit housing development organization, and her own research firm.

Before organizing and providing care for her mother, Karofsky filled interim positions for a statewide women's network—focusing on elder economic security—and for a coalition of state aging groups. She has written on institutional investing in seniors housing. Serving on nonprofit and municipal boards, she participates in policy discussions on demographic trends, affordable housing, and urban growth.

Karofsky holds an A.B. cum laude from Bryn Mawr College (economics) and master's degrees from Brandeis University (American history) and the University of Wisconsin-Madison (business). She completed eight marathons, several half-marathons, and countless 10K races. An only child, the mother of three, and grandmother of five, she lives in Madison.